GW00686326

MAKING SENSE OF OBSTETRIC DOPPLER ULTRASOUND

All clinical images used in this publication were obtained using Acuson ultrasound products from Siemens

MAKING SENSE OF OBSTETRIC DOPPLER ULTRASOUND

A HANDS-ON GUIDE

Christoph Lees
Consultant in Obstetrics and Fetal-Maternal Medicine,
The Rosie Maternity Hospital, Addenbrookes NHS Trust, Cambridge, UK

Colin Deane
Clinical Scientist, Department of Medical Engineering and Physics,
King's College Hospital, London, UK

Gerard Albaiges
Specialist in Obstetrics and Gynecology, Feto-Maternal Medicine Unit,
Hospital Joan XXIII, Tarragona, Spain

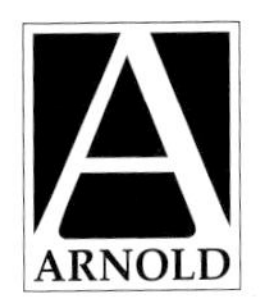

A member of the Hodder Headline Group
LONDON

First published in Great Britain in 2003 by
Arnold, a member of the Hodder Headline Group,
338 Euston Road, London NW1 3BH

http://www.hoddereducation.com

Distributed in the United States of America by Oxford University Press Inc.,
198 Madison Avenue, New York, NY10016
Oxford is a registered trademark of Oxford University Press

British Library Cataloguing in Publication Data
A catalogue record for this book is available from the British Library

Library of Congress Cataloging-in-Publication Data
A catalog record for this book is available from the Library of Congress

ISBN–10: 0 340 80919 1
ISBN–13: 978 0 340 80919 8

2 3 4 5 6 7 8 9 10

Commissioning Editor: Joanna Koster
Production Editor: Anke Ueberberg
Production Controller: Bryan Eccleshall
Cover Design: Terry Griffiths

Typeset in 10 on 12pt Clearface by Phoenix Photosetting, Chatham, Kent
Printed and bound in Italy.

CONTENTS

FOREWORD

Over the last half century, ultrasound imaging has created a revolution in the practice of obstetrics. This advance has enabled us to visualize and study the mother and fetus, facilitating many new diagnostic and therapeutic modalities. These advances were made possible by two pioneers.

Regius Professor of Midwifery, Ian Donald of Glasgow University, developed the first medical ultrasound scanning device 'using knowledge of radar from my days in the RAF'. Donald's ingenuity opened the secrets of the uterus. Sonography provided the means to study fetal anatomy, growth and development, amniotic fluid volume and placental pathology. Soon realtime was added to the instruments, and fetal motion could be visualized, enabling studies of fetal motion, heart function and fetal physiology.

In 1842 Christian Doppler, a physics professor at the University of Vienna, postulated that the apparent frequency of light or sound waves depends on the relative motion of the wave source and the observer. The Doppler principle, as we know it today, means that movement of a reflecting object toward the sound source results in an apparent increase in the frequency of the reflected sound, and movement away from the source results in a decrease. An instrument employing the Doppler principle was first used in obstetrics to listen to the fetal heart. Then it was employed in conjunction with electronic fetal heart rate monitoring instruments. The marriage of this technology to ultrasound imaging capability provided an exciting new technology, Doppler ultrasound, which is described in this book.

By identifying anatomical targets with imaging and measuring motion with Doppler, an enormous amount of valuable information can be gained about a pregnancy. Now we evaluate such things as the fetal heart anatomy and function, measure changes in blood flow in specific blood vessels, and study fetal respirations. Obviously, this modality has enabled a myriad of new studies in fetal physiology and pathophysiology.

Making Sense of Obstetric Doppler Ultrasound is a hands-on guide to skillful use of obstetric Doppler ultrasound. The authors have a talent for presenting material in a clear, concise, and practical manner. Complex concepts are made simple and logical, and the physics and safety of ultrasound are clearly presented. They provide excellent tutelage in developing optimal imaging and present illustrative case histories.

Personally, I can't stand to read instruction manuals. The time display on my VCR is still blinking. This hands-on guide is different because it is easy to read, and the illustrations are clear and helpful. The book will be a very valuable resource for anyone who wishes to enter the complex world of obstetric Doppler ultrasound painlessly. Congratulations to the authors.

John T Queenan MD
Professor and Chairman, Emeritus
Department of Obstetrics and Gynecology
Georgetown University Medical Center
Washington, DC, USA

1

DOPPLER ULTRASOUND – BASICS

Doppler ultrasound is widely used to investigate the human circulation. Practiced properly it is a reliable, reproducible and safe means to image and make measurements of normal and abnormal flow in arteries and veins.

Obstetric applications of Doppler pose particular challenges for ultrasound users. Fetal vessels are small, movement of the fetus can make accurate location of vessels difficult, and the rapid fetal heart rate requires fast imaging. Image clarity is highly dependent on the skill of the ultrasound operator. Operators need to understand how the images are produced and what changes they can make in their scanning to optimize the image and enable precise and accurate measurements to be made.

The first four chapters of this book explain how to produce good-quality pulsed wave and color-flow Doppler images safely in a logical manner, as follows:

- How Doppler images are formed
- Optimizing Doppler images
- Doppler measurements
- Safety of Doppler ultrasound

HOW DOPPLER IMAGES ARE FORMED

In ultrasound scanners, color-flow and pulsed-wave Doppler images are obtained from measurements of movement. A series of pulses is transmitted along a beam. The echoes from stationary tissue are the same from one pulse to the next. Echoes from moving scatterers, for example blood, show slight differences in time. The principles are illustrated in Fig. 1.1.

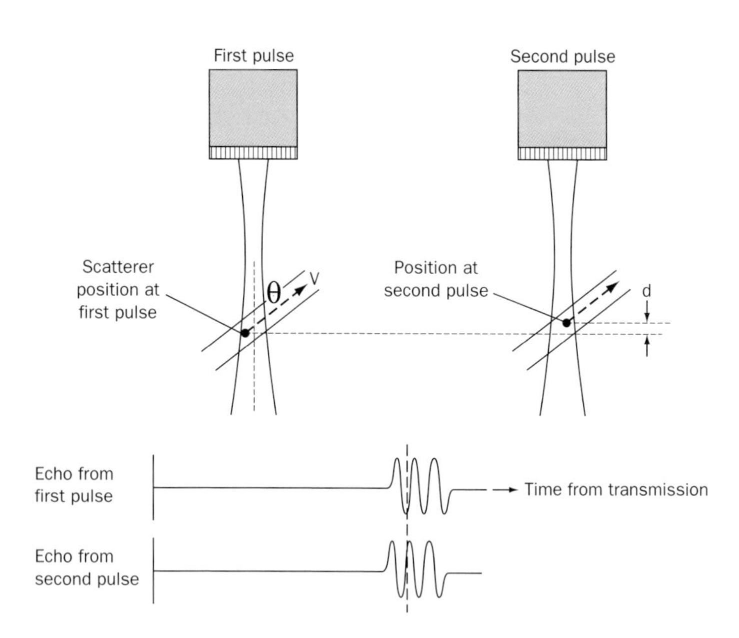

Figure 1.1 As blood moves through an ultrasound beam (*V*), the position of scatterers within it relative to the transducer changes. The echo from the second pulse returns slightly earlier than it did for the first pulse. The difference in time is used to measure the distance moved and from this the velocity is obtained.

In the diagram, the ultrasound scanner sends two pulses along a beam. If there are any moving scatterers passing through the beam, the transmit-to-receive time from the scatterers is slightly different in the second pulse. The difference in time is dependent on the distance moved in the direction of the beam. Since we know how frequently the pulses are sent out, the velocity of the scatterers in the direction of the beam can be calculated.

For pulsed-wave Doppler and the majority of color-flow imaging techniques, measurement of velocity is achieved by measurement of the change in phase in the returning echoes from blood at a particular time after transmission. This produces a Doppler frequency described in the well-known equation (Fig. 1.2):

$$\text{Doppler frequency} = f_d = \frac{2\,V f_t \cos\theta}{c}$$

where f_t is the transmitted ultrasound frequency, V is the velocity of the blood, θ is the angle between the beam and the direction of flow, and c is the speed of sound in tissue. A detailed explanation of how the Doppler equation is derived is given in Appendix A.

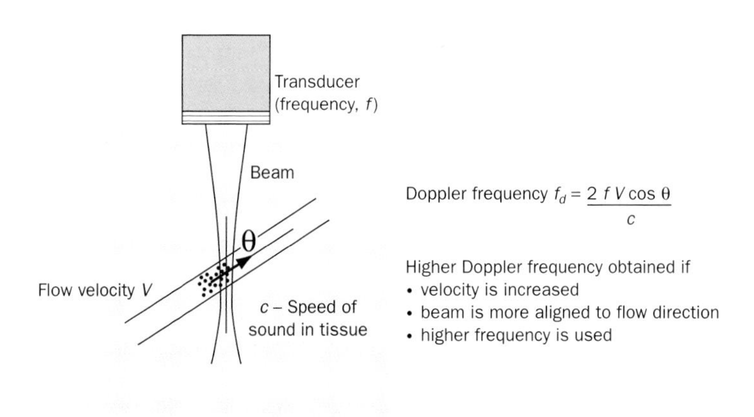

Figure 1.2 Factors affecting the Doppler frequency. The signal is dependent on the velocity of the blood, the transducer frequency and the angle between the vessel and the ultrasound beam.

The Doppler frequency determines the color-flow signal or Doppler spectrum. The equation shows us that the Doppler frequency is dependent on:

- Blood velocity. As velocity increases so does the Doppler frequency
- The beam/flow angle. The Doppler frequency increases as the beam is more aligned to the flow. As can be appreciated from Fig. 1.1 and the Doppler equation, there is very little signal at angles close to 90°
- Ultrasound frequency. Higher ultrasound frequencies give increased Doppler frequencies; however, as for ultrasound generally, lower ultrasound frequencies have better penetration in tissue. The frequency used is a compromise between sensitivity to low flows and adequate penetration

DOPPLER MODES, PULSED-WAVE DOPPLER, COLOR-FLOW IMAGING AND POWER DOPPLER

Doppler methods are a measure of **velocity** in the direction of the ultrasound beam from which the color-flow and Doppler spectrum displays are produced. The requirements of color-flow imaging (including power Doppler) and pulsed-wave Doppler are very different. The pulses and signal processing used for these modes are optimized for each. In practice, color-flow imaging and pulsed-wave Doppler complement each other and are used in conjunction with each other in an ultrasound examination. Figure 1.3 shows an ultrasound image combining B-mode, color-flow imaging and pulsed-wave Doppler with the major features described.

The basic characteristics of each mode are described in Table 1.1.

Basics of Color-flow Imaging

In color-flow imaging, a region of the image is investigated for flow. Velocity vectors over the area are calculated and vessels are displayed as color images over the B-mode image. Colors used are usually red and blue to indicate flow towards and away from the beam direction; the operator may choose which (Fig. 1.4).

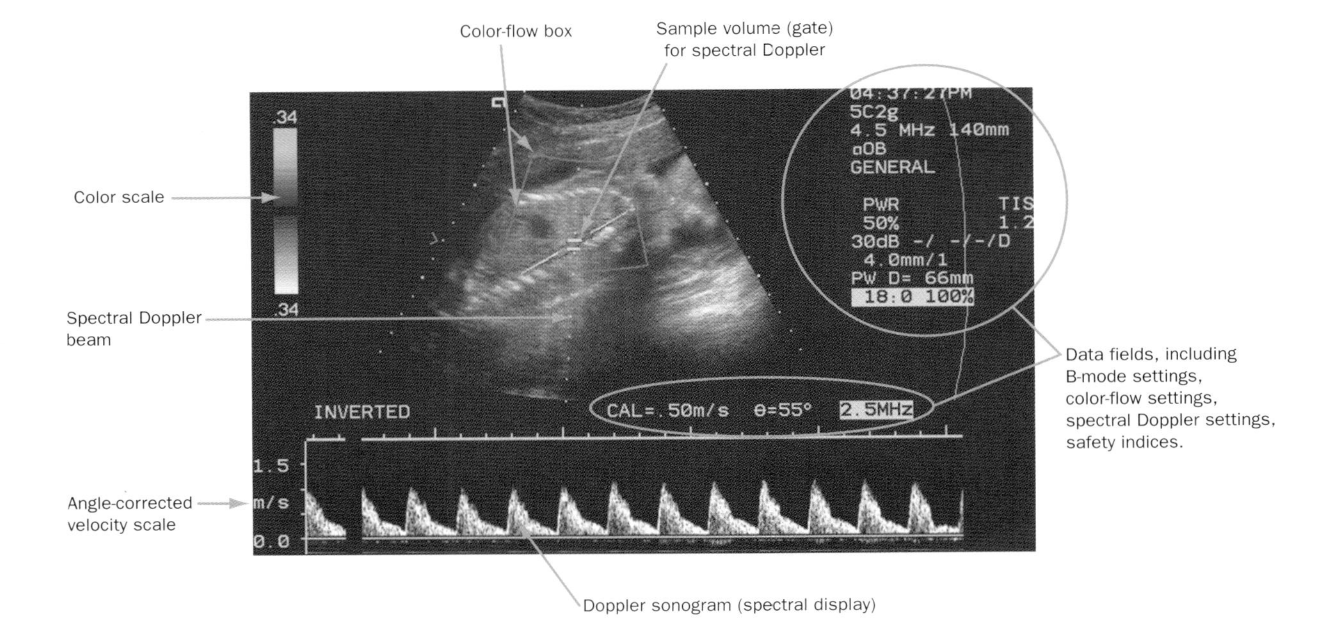

Figure 1.3 Image of a fetal aorta showing B-mode, color-flow imaging and spectral Doppler sonogram.

Table 1.1 The basic characteristics of pulsed-wave Doppler, color-flow imaging and power Doppler

Color-flow imaging
- Produces a color map of flow over a region of the image
- Limited flow information – the color shows the mean velocity vector at each point (vector – velocity in the direction of the beam)
- Limited temporal resolution – because of the need to sample over a large area, flow images are usually updated at a lower frame rate than B-mode for the same image area
- Moderate spatial resolution. Pulses are longer than for B-mode so axial resolution is not as good. The lateral resolution is usually not as good as for B-mode because of the use of a lower line density

Pulsed-wave Doppler (also described as spectral Doppler)
- Examines flow at one site
- Gives an analysis of the distribution of flow velocities in the sample volume
- Gives a detailed analysis of the time variation of flow (temporal resolution) – the flow waveform
- Allows calculation of velocity and flow waveform indices
- Limited spatial resolution (minimum sample volume size typically 1–1.5 mm)

Power Doppler (also described as Doppler energy; amplitude Doppler)
- Similar to color-flow imaging. Directional information is usually sacrificed and temporal resolution is reduced to gain better sensitivity to low flows and low velocities

There are many different color maps available, some of which use different hues and saturations of color to indicate increased velocities. The color depicted is dependent on the beam/vessel angle. This can lead to a range of colors in a vessel as it changes direction through a region of the image. The geometry of the beams in an image (for example in a curvilinear array) may itself lead to changes in beam vessel angle throughout the display. When the angle is close to 90° there may be little or no color displayed (Fig. 1.5).

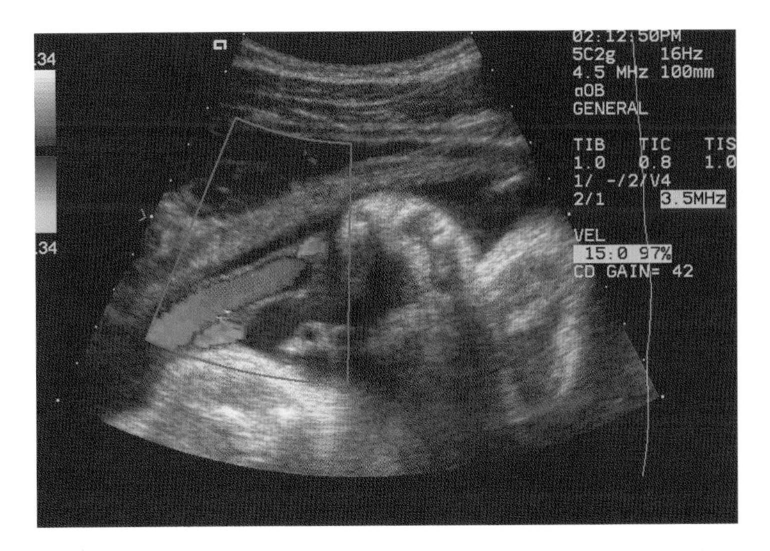

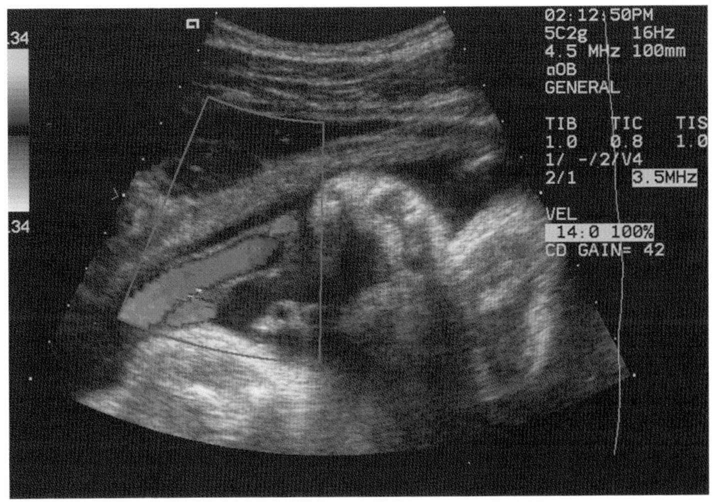

Figure 1.4 Image of umbilical arteries and vein. The color display shows the direction of flow with flow towards the transducer, coded red (top). The color assignment can be reversed (bottom).

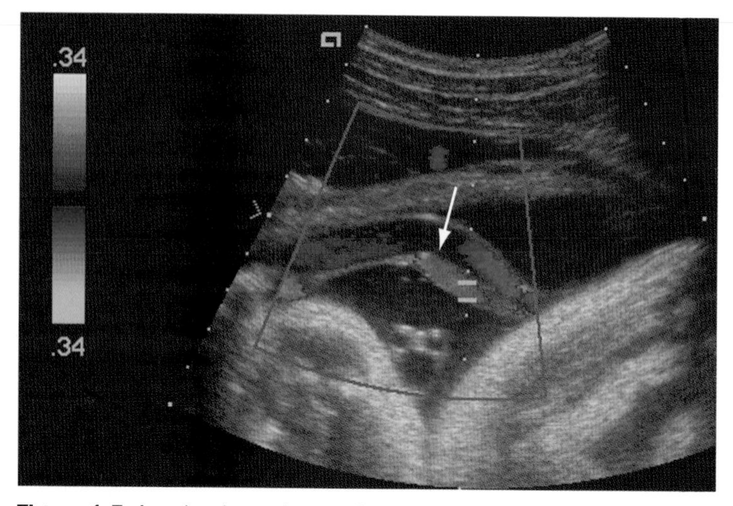

Figure 1.5 Angular dependence of color-flow imaging. As the flow/beam angle passes through 90°, no color flow is displayed (arrow).

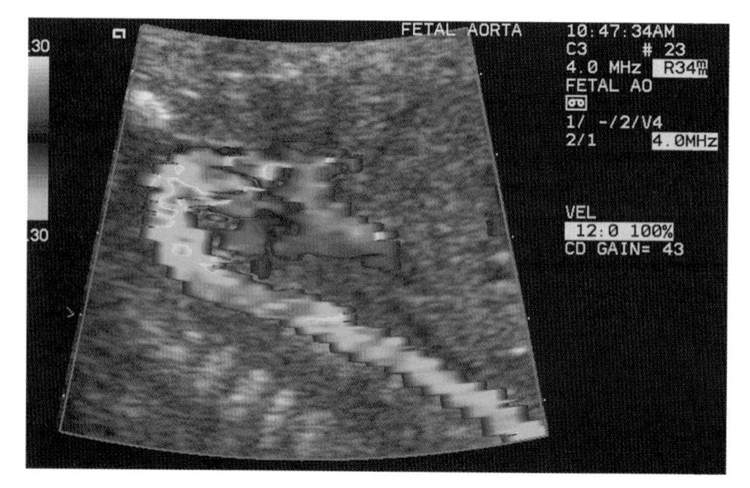

Figure 1.6 Color image of a fetal aorta. With the image zoomed, the limited axial and lateral resolution results in a stepped appearance of the color image.

To obtain color-flow images, the scanner needs to send several pulses (typically four to six) along each line to detect relative movement. In order to maintain an adequate frame rate, the line density in the color image is not as high as in B-mode. The color pulses are longer and usually have a higher amplitude than the B-mode pulses. These factors have important consequences for color-flow imaging:

- The frame rate for the color-flow image may not be as high as for B-mode alone
- The spatial resolution of the color image is not as good as for B-mode (Fig. 1.6)
- The ultrasound acoustic output is usually higher for color-flow imaging than for B-mode, which has implications for safe scanning practice (see Chapter 4).

Basics of Pulsed-wave Doppler

For pulsed-wave Doppler, a sample volume is placed on a specific part of the vessel under investigation and a sonogram is obtained. Figure 1.7 shows the components of the sonogram. Because the ultrasound is concentrated on one location, the sonogram can be updated many times (around 100) per second and displays the range and distribution of velocities in the sample volume as they change in real time. The sonogram shows the Doppler frequencies measured and, as in the color-flow image, it is highly dependent on the beam/vessel angle. The relationship is shown diagrammatically in Fig. 1.8. At angles close to 90° there is little flow signal. With the flow away from the transducer there is an inverted sonogram although this can be re-inverted on the display by the operator.

The sonogram permits measurements of flow characteristics. The shape of the flow waveform is itself often very useful and it is not always necessary to try to measure true velocities. To measure true velocities, an angle correction must be made between the beam and the vessel. Without an angle correction the velocities, although displayed, may be incorrect (Fig. 1.9).

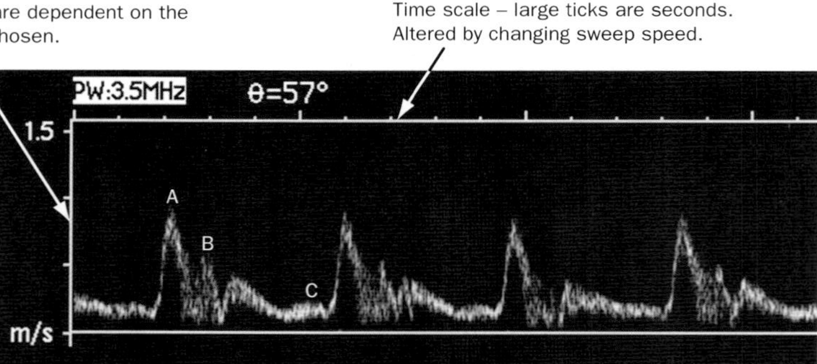

PW:3.5MHz
θ=57°
1.5
m/s
A
B
C

The velocity/frequency scale shows the range of velocities/frequencies in the flow waveform. The scale is dependent on the pulse repetition frequency/scale used. In duplex scanning, the velocity values on it are dependent on the beam/vessel angle chosen.
Time scale – large ticks are seconds. Altered by changing sweep speed.
The Doppler spectrum shows
• the range of velocities at every point in time (given by the height of sonogram)
• the distribution of velocities (given by the intensity of the sonogram)
e.g. the velocities at A are higher than B and lowest at C.
At C there is a brighter sonogram than at B, suggesting more uniform velocities at C.
There appears to be more spectral broadening at B than at C.

Figure 1.7 The Doppler sonogram.

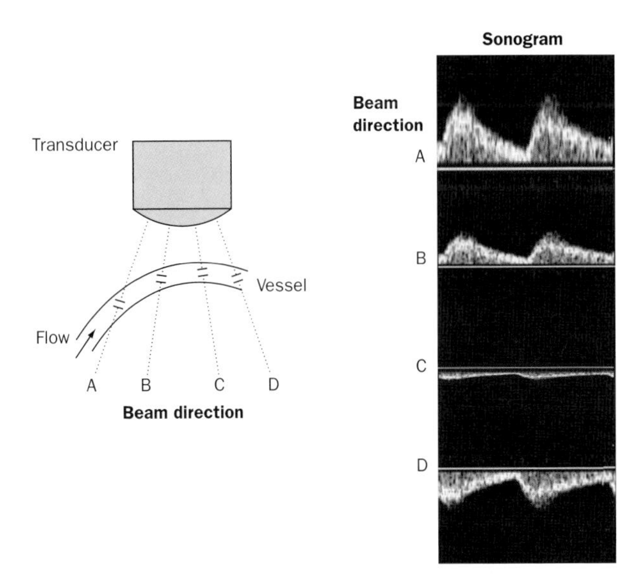

Figure 1.8 Angular dependence of the Doppler spectrum. The height and direction of the sonogram is altered as the beam/vessel angle changes.

Scale and Aliasing

One of the main controls used to alter the appearance of the color-flow and pulsed-wave image is the scale. This controls how frequently pulses are emitted to detect movement. If the blood is moving slowly, the operator should choose a low scale so that pulses are transmitted less frequently (i.e. a low pulse repetition frequency, PRF) to detect the small amount of movement between pulses. If the blood is moving more quickly, the scale should be increased so that pulses are transmitted at a higher PRF.

If a low scale/low PRF is used for high velocities, an effect known as aliasing can occur. In aliasing, high velocities are misrepresented as low or reverse velocities. The reason for aliasing is described in Appendix A. The effects are shown for color-flow imaging in Fig. 1.10 and for pulsed-wave Doppler in Fig. 1.11.

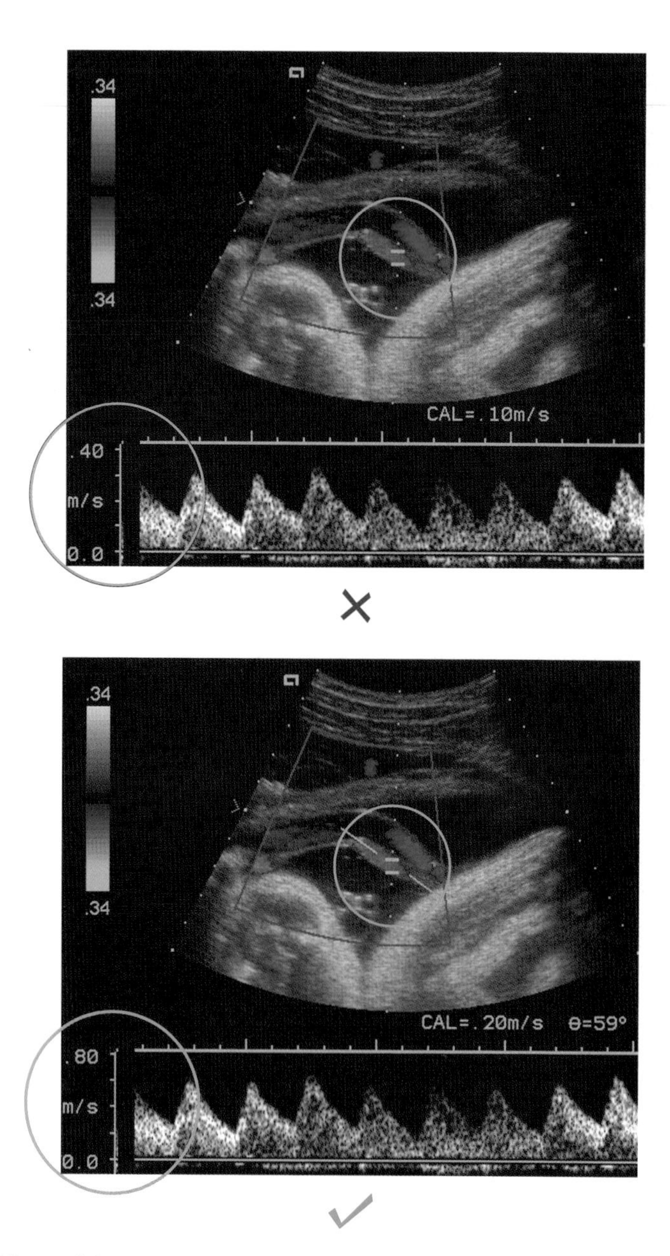

Figure 1.9 Beam/vessel angle correction. When no angle correction is made, the velocities displayed are incorrect (top). The true velocities are displayed when the angle correction is made correctly (bottom).

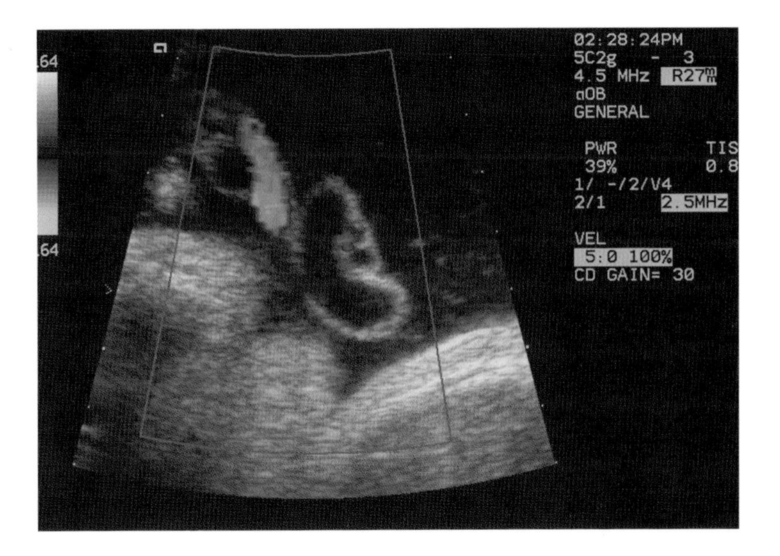

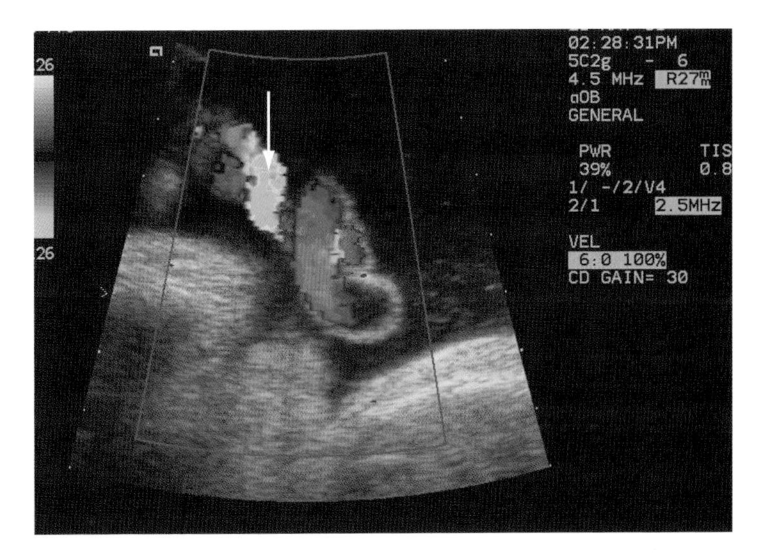

Figure 1.10 Color flow of umbilical vein and artery. With the color scale set high (top) no flow is detected in the vein but the higher velocities in an artery are displayed. With the color scale set low (bottom) flow is detected in the vein but aliasing occurs in the artery (arrow).

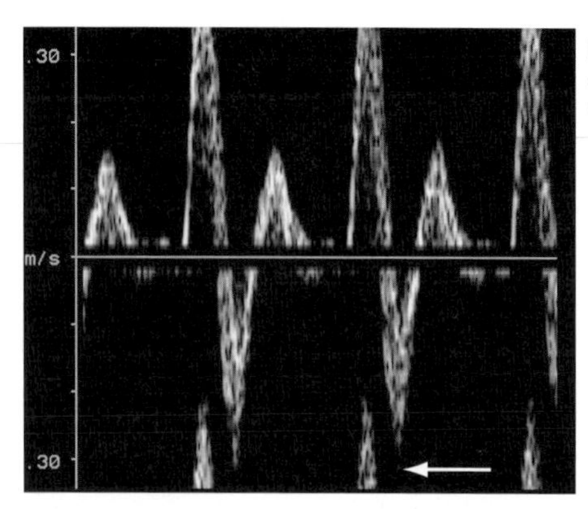

Peak systolic velocities appear as reverse flow (arrow)

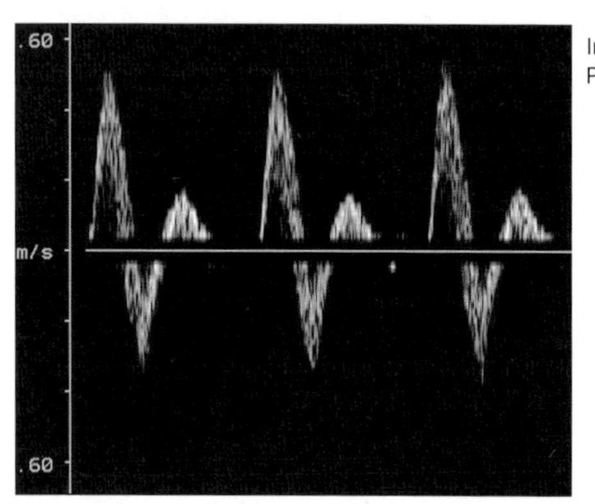

Increasing scale/PRF makes PSV unambiguous

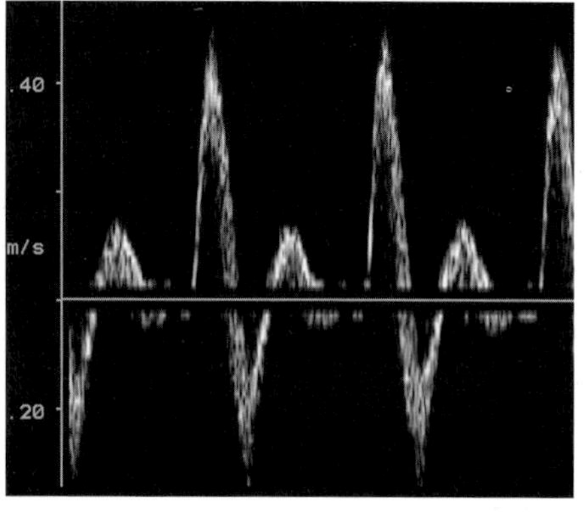

Lowering baseline allows PSV to appear as forward flow

Figure 1.11 Aliasing in spectral Doppler. With the velocity scale set too low, the peak systolic velocities are displayed incorrectly. This can be corrected by altering the baseline or increasing the scale. (PRF, pulse repetition frequency; PSV, peak systolic velocity).

Power Doppler

Power Doppler shows the amplitude of the color-flow signal rather than the frequency change. The amplitude varies little with flow velocity and direction and so the image shows a consistent view of vasculature in the image plane but without directional or velocity information (Fig. 1.12). The consistency of signal allows the use of image-processing techniques that make power Doppler sensitive to low flows and velocities.

Duplex and Triplex Scanning

The different requirements of B-mode, color-flow imaging and pulsed-wave Doppler mean that when two or more modes are used simultaneously, the performance of each is constrained by the amount of time available. Manufacturers make various compromises to allow acceptable images in each mode. For

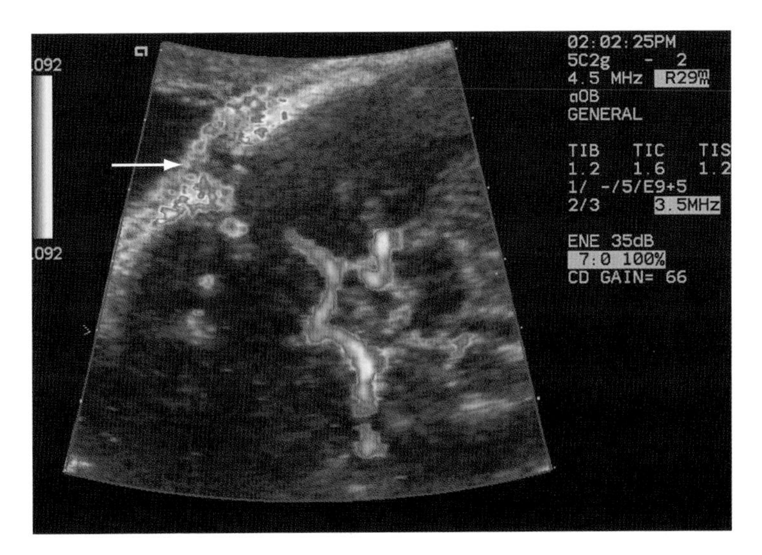

Figure 1.12 Power Doppler image of a fetal circle of Willis. The direction of flow is not displayed but there is good sensitivity to flow in the major vessels. Note the extraneous signals at the skull surface (arrow).

example, when the pulsed-wave Doppler is used, the image and color-flow image is usually frozen so that a good-quality sonogram can be obtained.

Some manufacturers offer a 'triplex' facility whereby B-mode, color-flow imaging and pulsed-wave Doppler all run concurrently. For the operator, this has the advantage of allowing them to see if a vessel changes position in an image. However, this may result in serious compromises, for example in image spatial resolution, frame rate, pulsed-wave Doppler resolution, and maximum velocity measurable.

FURTHER READING

Evans DH, McDicken WN (2000) *Doppler Ultrasound: Physics and Instrumentation*, 2nd edn. Chichester: Wiley.

2

OPTIMIZING DOPPLER IMAGES

The diagnostic potential of Doppler ultrasound images is dependent on image quality. As in B-mode, there are several factors and controls that affect the appearance of Doppler images. This chapter describes these factors and suggests ways to optimize images.

COLOR-FLOW IMAGING

The factors that influence the appearance of the color image are listed in Table 2.1. Most of these can be preprogrammed into a specific application setting. By selecting that specific application (for example, first trimester, second trimester or fetal cardiac), the controls are set appropriately to begin scanning. Applications specialists from ultrasound companies can help in choosing settings for specific applications.

Many of these factors (including filter, post-processing, and preprocessing settings) may not need to be changed during an examination. However, the major controls (see below) can make large differences to image appearance and do need to be optimized throughout the scan.

The probe should be placed so that the vessels under investigation are aligned towards the beam. Beam/vessel angles close to 90° produce poor Doppler images (Fig. 2.1).

Table 2.1 Settings affecting color-flow images

Main factors

- Power: transmitted power into tissue
  Gain: overall sensitivity to flow signals
- Transmission frequency: trades penetration for sensitivity and resolution
- Pulse repetition frequency (PRF, also called scale):
  Low PRF to look at low velocities
  High PRF reduces aliasing at high velocities
- Area of investigation: larger area reduces frame rate and spatial resolution
- Focus: color-flow image optimized at focal zone

Other factors

- Triplex: color PRF and frame rate reduced by need for B-mode/pulsed-wave pulses
- Persistence: high persistence produces smoother image but reduces temporal resolution
- Pre-processing: trades resolution against frame rate
- Filter: high filter cuts out more noise but more of flow signal
- Post-processing: assigning color map/variance

Once the image is aligned, the major controls are optimized to improve the appearance of the image. These are:

- Power and gain. Color flow uses higher intensity than B-mode so it is important to pay attention to safety indices (see Chapter 4). Power and gain should be set to obtain good signals with little extraneous signal from surrounding tissue (Fig. 2.2)
- Frequency selection. Many transducers can operate at several frequencies. High frequencies give better sensitivity to low flow and have better spatial resolution; low frequencies have better penetration (Fig. 2.3) and are less susceptible to aliasing at high velocities
- Velocity scale/pulse repetition frequency (PRF). Low PRFs should be used to look at low velocities but aliasing may occur if high velocities are encountered (see Fig. 1.10)

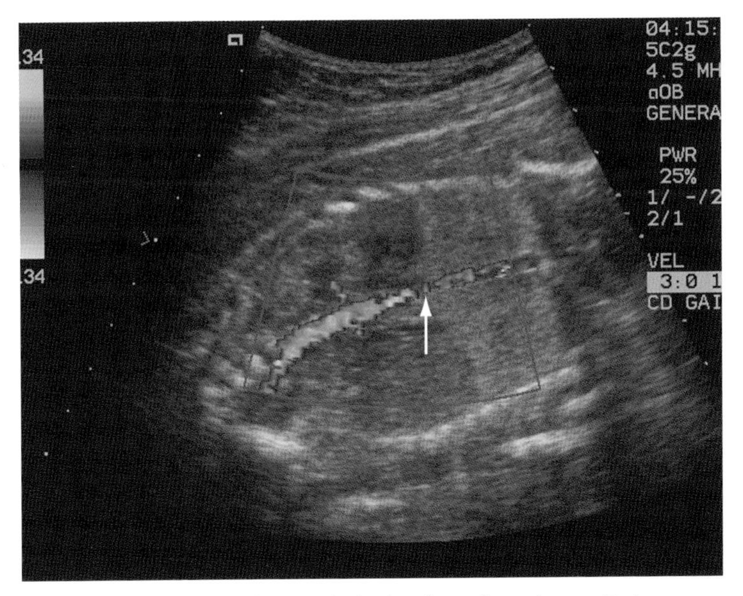

Figure 2.1 Poor beam/flow angle in the thoracic aorta results in a poor color image (arrow). The lower abdominal aorta is better displayed because it is better aligned to beam direction.

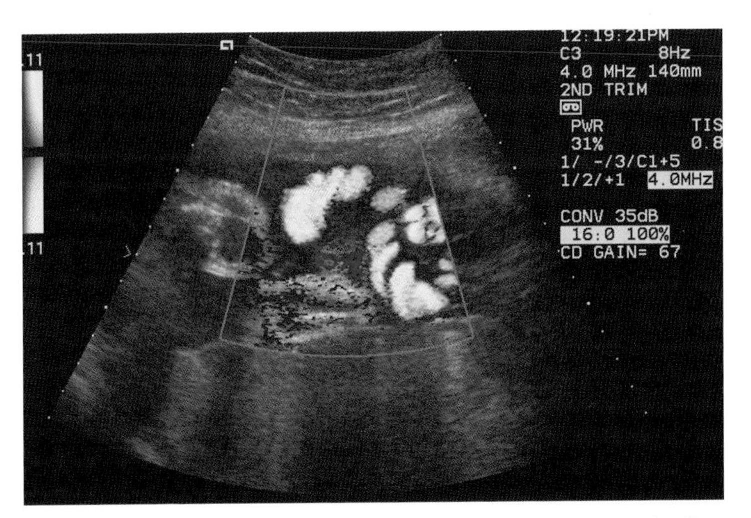

Figure 2.2 The color gain is too high and there is extraneous color-flow signal from tissue.

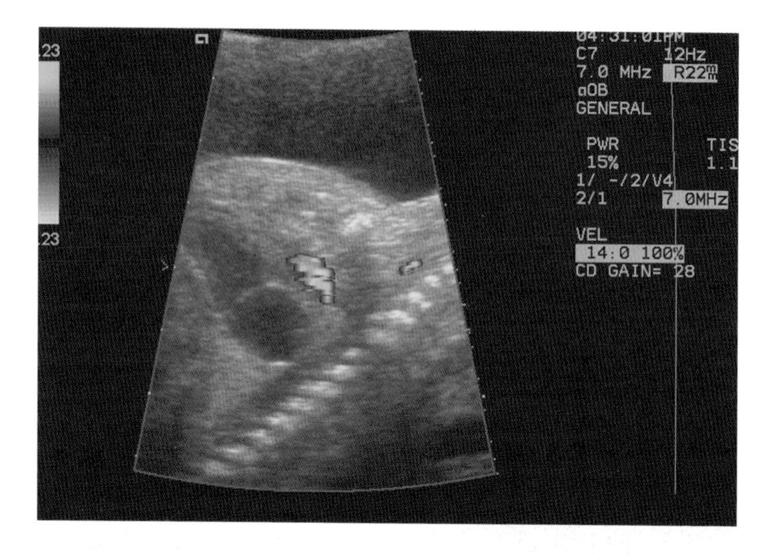

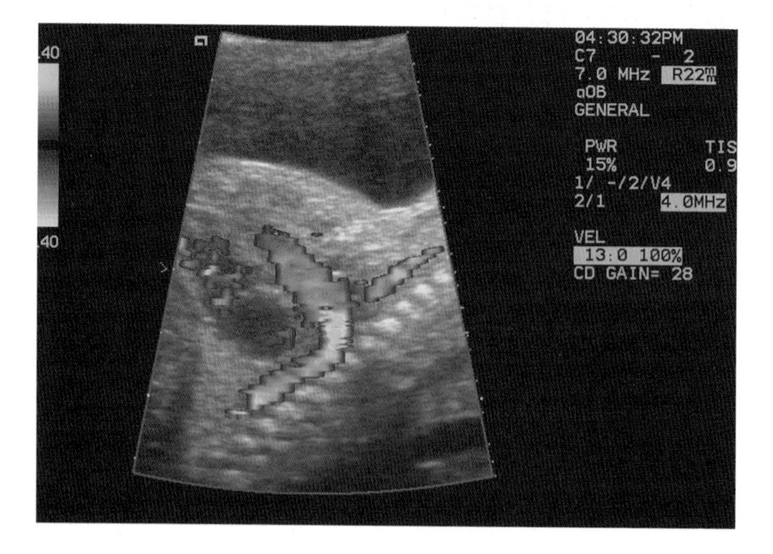

Figure 2.3 Effect of transmission frequency on the color-flow image. With identical power and gain settings, the 7 MHz color-flow image produces poor filling of the heart and aorta (top) when compared with 4 MHz image (bottom).

- Focus. Make sure the focus is at the level of the area of interest. This can make a significant difference to the appearance and accuracy of the image (Fig. 2.4)

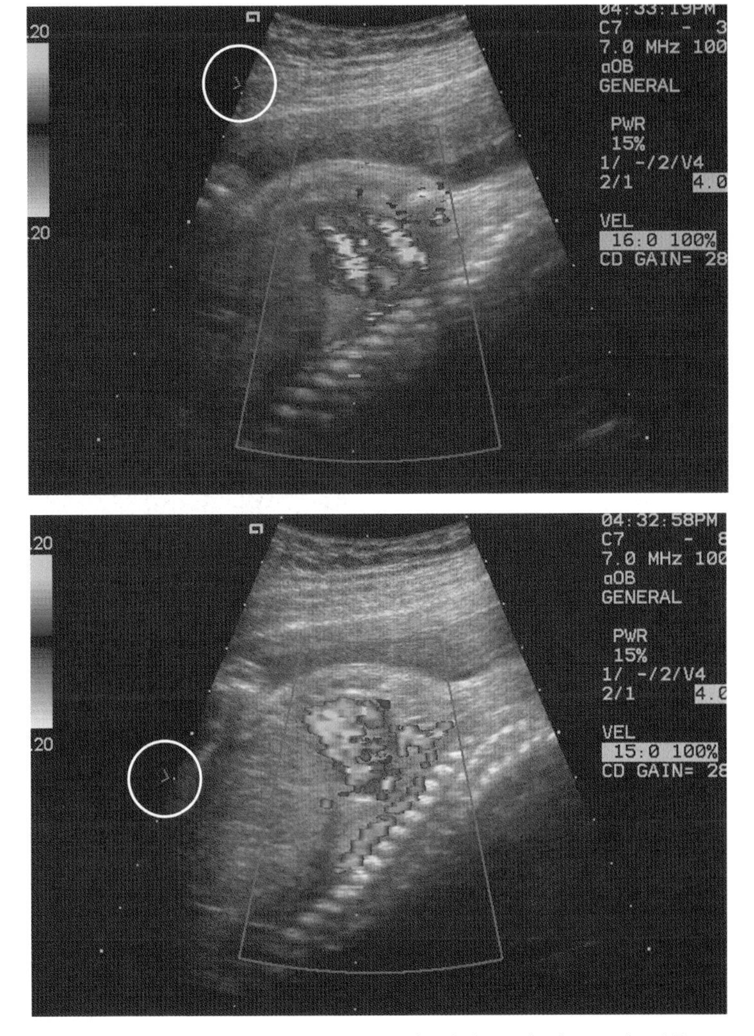

Figure 2.4 With the focus set too high (top) the color image (and B-mode) is poorly displayed. The image is clearer with the focus set to the region of interest (bottom).

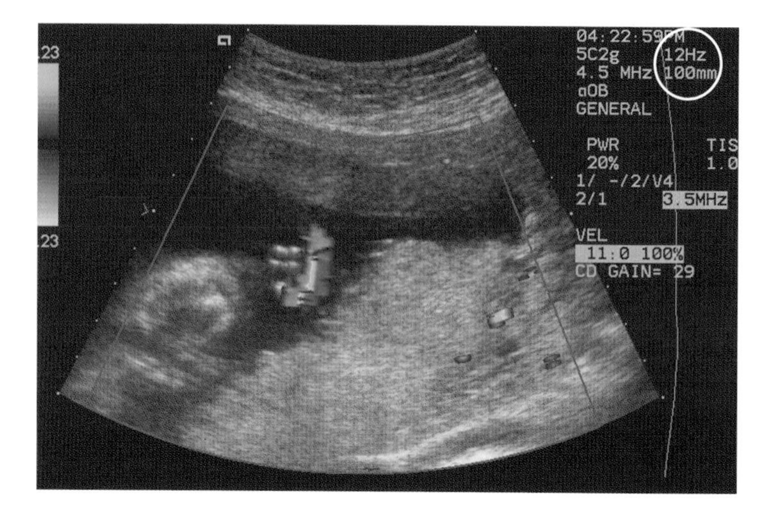

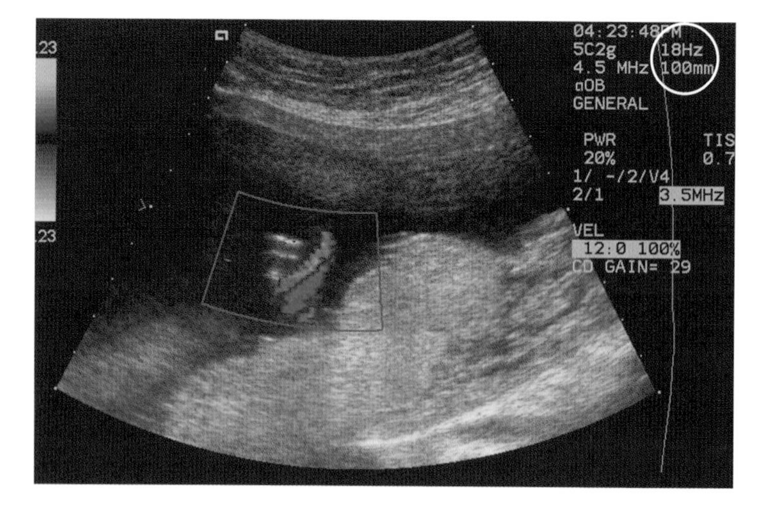

Figure 2.5 With a large color box (top), the frame rate is low (12 fps, white circle) and the umbilical artery and veins are not clearly defined. With a small color box (bottom), the frame rate increases and the improved spatial resolution results in improved definition of the artery and vein.

- Region of interest. Because more pulses are needed for color-flow imaging than for B-mode, reducing the width and maximum depth of the color-flow area under investigation can improve frame rate and spatial resolution (Fig. 2.5)

Practical guidelines for color-flow imaging are summarized in Table 2.2.

Table 2.2 Practical guidelines for color-flow imaging

1	Select the appropriate applications/set-up key: this optimizes parameters for specific examinations.
2	Set power to within study limits and adjust gain to optimize the color signal
3	Use probe positioning/beam steering to obtain satisfactory beam/vessel angle
4	Ensure focus is at the region of interest
5	Adjust pulse repetition frequency (PRF)/scale to suit the flow conditions: Low PRFs are more sensitive to low flows/velocities but may produce aliasing High PRFs reduce aliasing but are less sensitive to low velocities
6	Set the color flow region to appropriate size: A smaller color flow 'box' may lead to a better frame rate and better color resolution/sensitivity. Zooming the image to concentrate B-mode and color-flow image in a small area may have the same effect.

The factors influencing the power Doppler signal are similar to those for color-flow imaging, with the exception that aliasing does not occur because there is no measure of the velocity or direction of flow.

PULSED-WAVE DOPPLER IMAGING

The factors that influence the appearance of the Doppler spectrum are listed in Table 2.3. As with B-mode and color-flow imaging,

Table 2.3 Settings affecting pulsed-wave Doppler images

Main factors

- Power: transmitted power into tissue
- Gain: overall sensitivity to flow signals
- Pulse repetition frequency (PRF, also called scale):
  Low PRF to examine low-velocity flow
  High PRF reduces aliasing
- Gate size: determines how much of the vessel width is insonated
- Sweep: affects the appearance of the time scale of the sonogram
- Live duplex/triplex spectral resolution constrained by the need for B-mode/color pulses

Other factors

- Gate: sharpness of resolution
- Filter: high filter cuts out more noise but more of flow signal
- Postprocessing: assigns brightness to output

most of these can be preprogrammed into a specific application setting. Many of these factors may not need to be changed during an examination.

The probe should be placed so that the vessels under investigation are aligned towards the beam. Beam/vessel angles close to 90° produce poor Doppler images (Fig. 2.6) and will lead to unreliable measurements.

Once the image is aligned, the major controls are optimized to improve the appearance of the image. These controls are:

- Power and gain. Pulsed-wave Doppler uses higher intensity power than B-mode so it is important to pay attention to safety indices. Power and gain should be set so that clear signals are obtained (Fig. 2.7)
- Velocity scale/PRF. Low PRFs should be used to look at low velocities but aliasing may occur if high velocities are encountered (Fig. 2.8)

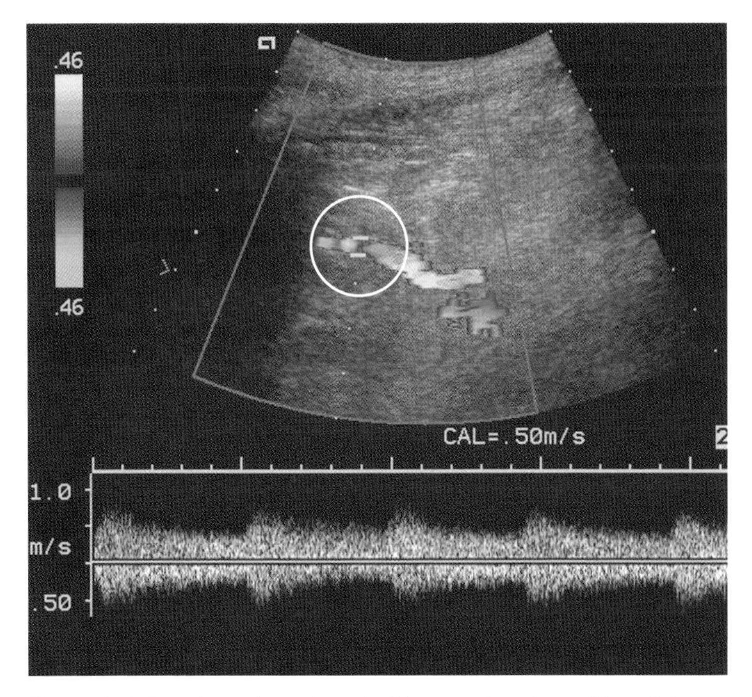

Figure 2.6 Poor beam/vessel angle. The sample volume (ringed) has been placed at a point where the angle between the beam and flow is nearly 90°, and the sonogram is unclear.

- Gate size (sample volume). If flow measurements are being attempted, the whole vessel should be insonated. A large gate may include signals from adjacent vessels
- Sweep speed. Altering the sweep speed changes the appearance of the flow waveforms (Fig. 2.9). If the spectrum is too compressed, measurements may be difficult
- Angle correction. If measurements of velocity are to be made, the angle between the beam and vessel must be correctly adjusted (see Fig. 1.9). Angles of greater than 60° should not be used because of possible errors (see p. 29)

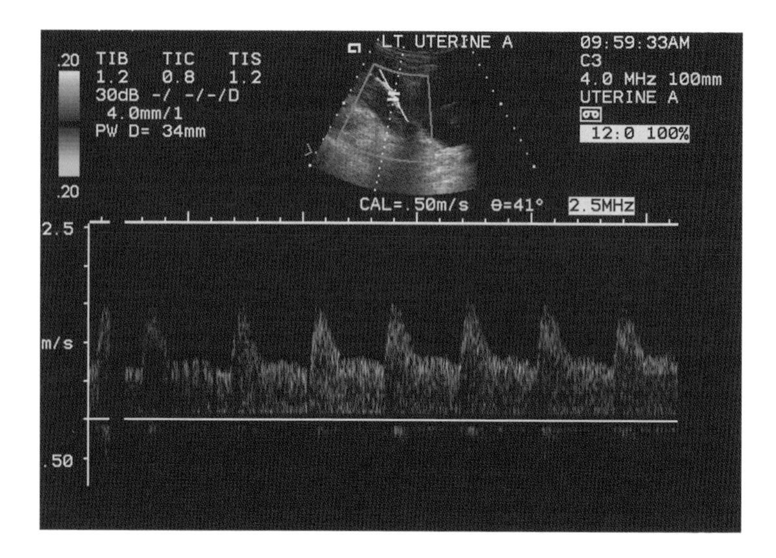

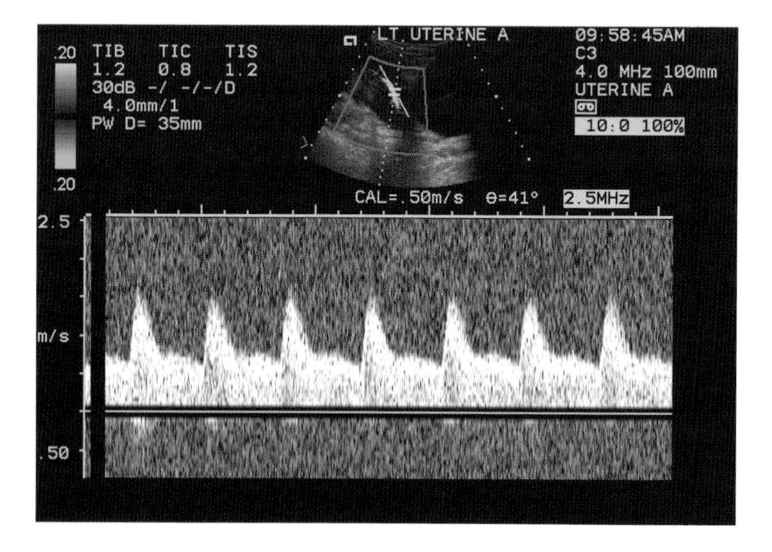

Figure 2.7 Incorrect gain settings. The gain is too low (top) and too high (bottom), leading to poor sonograms with possible errors in velocities displayed.

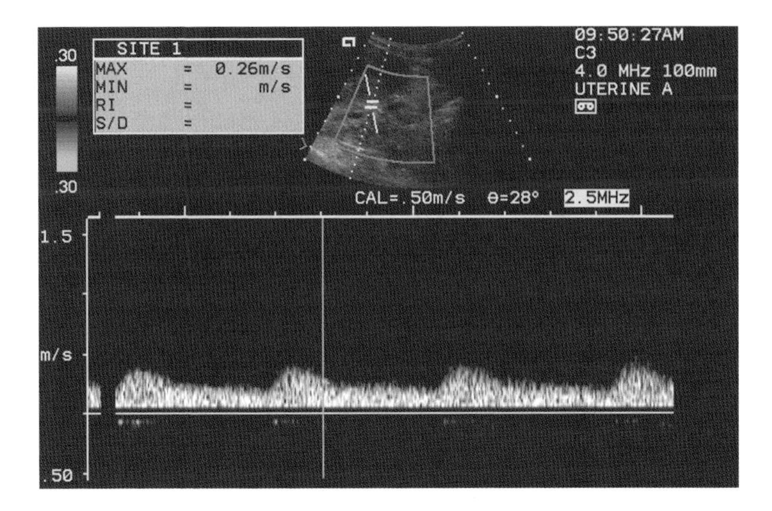

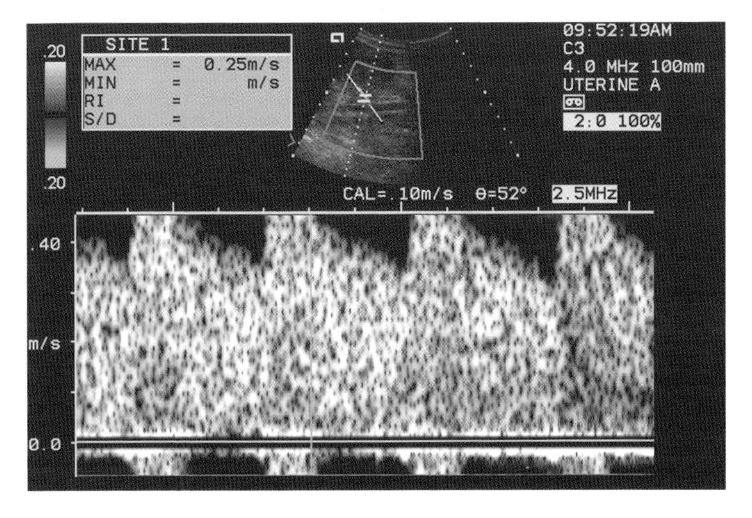

Figure 2.8 Incorrect scale settings. The scale is set too high (top) and too low (bottom). In both cases, the flow waveform shape is not clearly displayed.

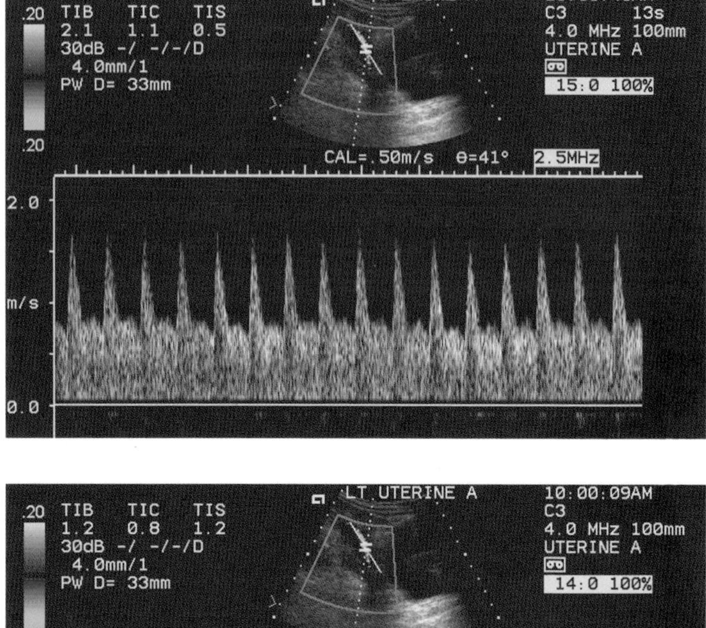

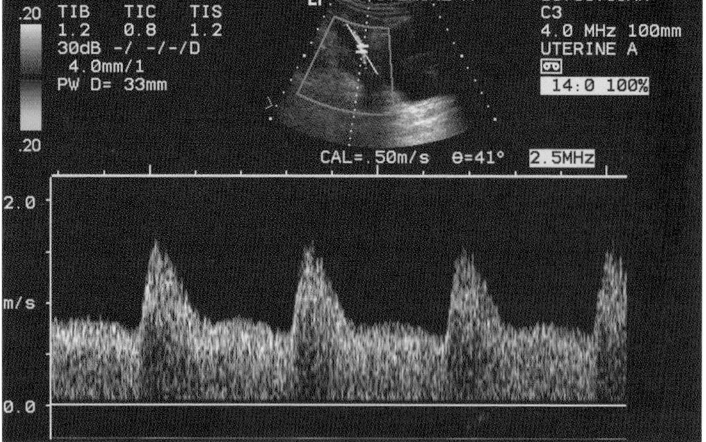

Figure 2.9 Sweep speed set too slow (top), makes it difficult to assess flow waveform shape. With the sweep speed increased (bottom), the sonogram displays the waveform shape clearly.

Table 2.4 Practical guidelines for pulsed-wave Doppler imaging

1	Set power to within fetal study limits
2	Position the pulsed-wave Doppler cursor on the vessel to be investigated
3	Adjust gain so that sonogram is clearly visible and free of noise
4	Use probe positioning/beam steering to obtain satisfactory beam/vessel angle. Angles close to 90° will give ambiguous/unclear values
5	Adjust PRF/scale and baseline to suit flow conditions Sonogram should be clear and not aliased
6	Adjust sweep speed to suit the heart rate
7	Set sample volume to correct size. Correct angle to obtain accurate velocities. Use the B-mode and color flow image of the vessel to make the angle correction.

Practical guidelines for pulsed-wave Doppler imaging are summarized in Table 2.4.

ANGLE CORRECTION AND VELOCITY ERRORS

The accuracy of the velocity measurements made depends on the accuracy of the beam/vessel angle correction. Inevitably, the operator makes errors because of the limited resolution of the image, inaccurate alignment on a curved vessel (e.g. umbilical artery) and errors in instrumentation. However, the effect of errors can be lessened if low beam/vessel angles are used.

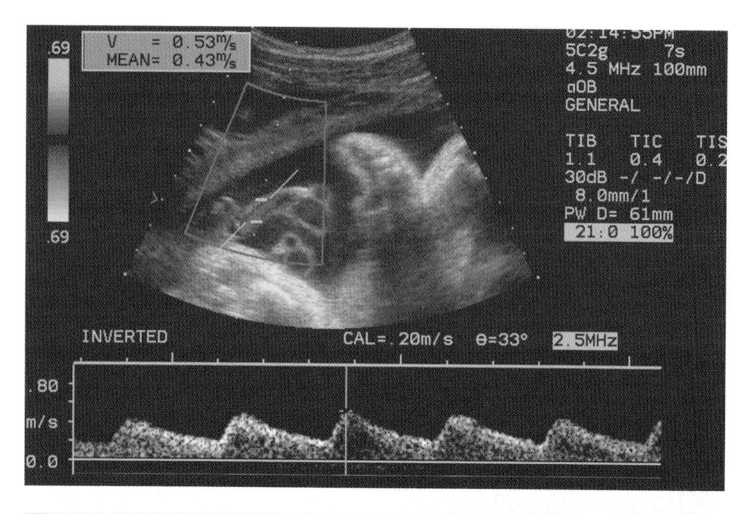

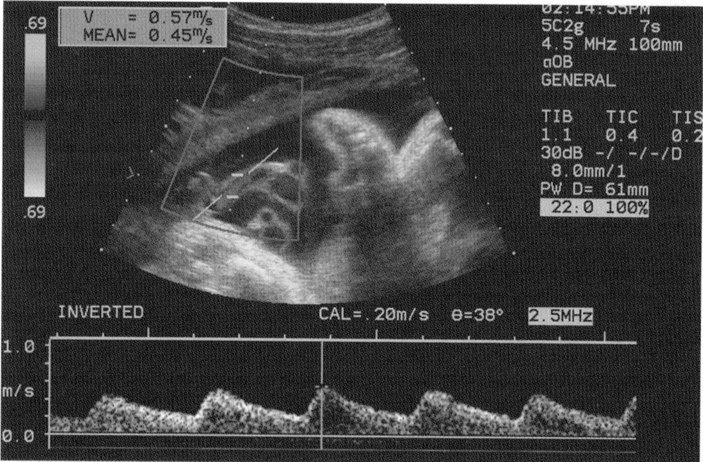

Figure 2.10 Peak systolic velocity with beam/vessel angle correction of 33° (top) and 38° (bottom). In both cases, the angle correction on the screen appears plausible.

Figure 2.10 shows the effect of a + 5° error when a beam/vessel angle of 33° is used. The measured peak systolic velocity rises from 53 cm/s to 57 cm/s, an error of 7.5%.

In Figure 2.11 the effects of the same 5° error are shown at 55°. Peak systolic velocity rises from 100 cm/s to 115 cm/s, an error of 15%.

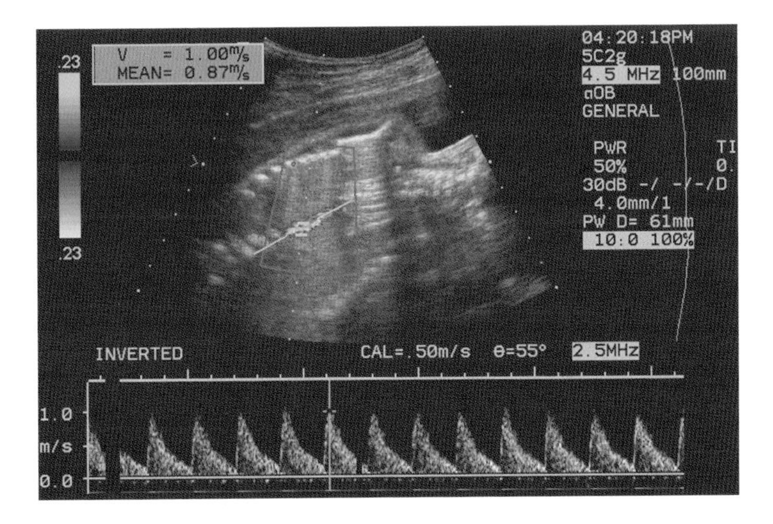

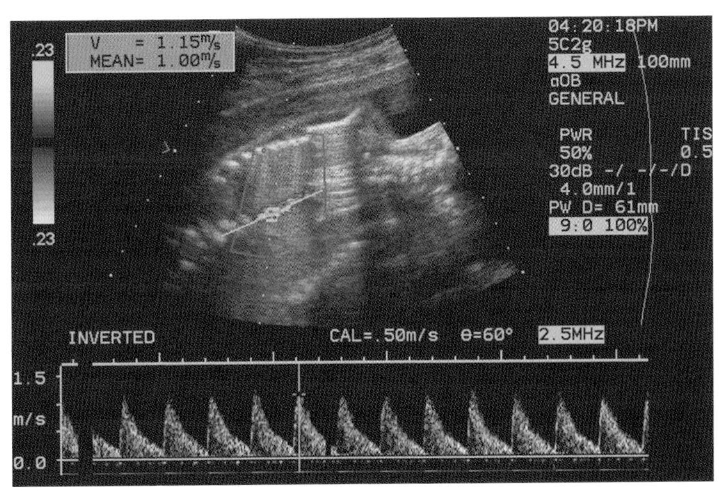

Figure 2.11 Peak systolic velocity with beam/vessel angle correction of 55° (top) and 60° (bottom). In both cases, the angle correction appears plausible.

Table 2.5 The percentage errors for a + 5° error in beam/vessel angle

Beam/vessel angle (degrees)	Percentage velocity error for a + 5° angle error
10	1
20	3
30	5
40	7
50	10
60	15
70	24
80	50

The percentage errors for a + 5° error in beam/vessel angle are listed for various angles in Table 2.5.

There are additional errors inherent in the use of arrays to produce the Doppler ultrasound beam. Again, errors increase with increasing beam/vessel angle. It is prudent not to use angles of greater than 60° if velocities are to be measured.

3

DOPPLER MEASUREMENTS

Color-flow and pulse-wave Doppler display blood velocity in the direction of the ultrasound beam. If an angle correction between the beam and vessel can be made, the true velocities in vessels are shown (see Fig. 1.9).

Doppler measurements of the circulation are usually made from the sonogram, which shows the distribution of velocities in the sample volume and the change in velocities over time (the flow waveform). Combined with measurements of vessel cross-section, velocity measurements can give a measure of volume flow, although this is fraught with possible errors and needs care.

FLOW WAVEFORMS AND FLOW PROFILES

It is important to distinguish between the terms flow waveforms and flow profiles.

The action of the heart causes pulsatile flow in large arteries. Flow in some veins is pulsatile as a result of the changing pressure in the right side of the heart opposing the flow. The flow waveform describes the changing flow with time. Arterial flow usually shows high systolic velocities with lower velocities in diastole. An example is shown in Fig. 3.1. There may be no flow in diastole if peripheral resistance is high. The shape of the flow waveform is

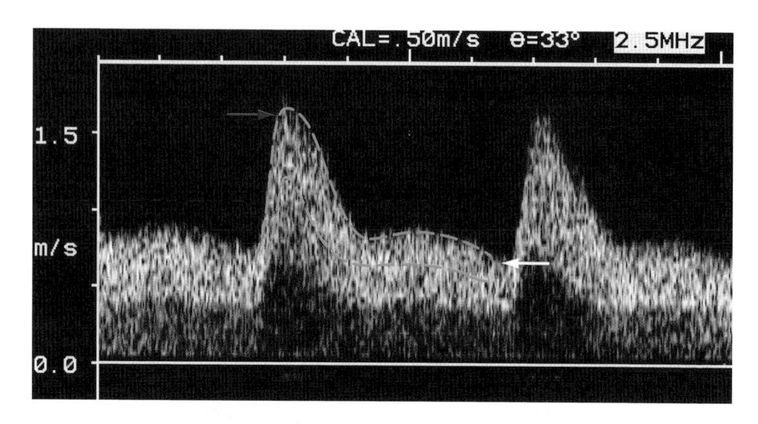

Figure 3.1 Velocity measurements from a sonogram. Orange line, time-averaged mean velocity (mean velocity in the volume sampled); blue line, time-averaged maximum velocity (maximum velocity over the period measured); red arrow, peak systolic velocity; white arrow, end-diastolic velocity.

dependent on many factors, but in specific vascular beds it may be predominantly dependent on distal resistance.

The flow profile describes the way velocities vary across a vessel at any time. Flow is slowest next to the vessel wall and is usually highest in the center of the vessel. The effect is sometimes observed in the color image of a vessel, although the small size of fetal vessels and the limited spatial resolution of color-flow imaging may obscure this. The flow profile results in a range of velocities being displayed in a sonogram, depending on how much of the vessel is insonated.

Under normal conditions, flow in vessels is described as laminar (i.e. blood moves as a series of adjacent laminae sliding over each other). The flow profile may be blunt or may approach or be parabolic in shape. The flow waveform influences the flow profile shape; for example, sudden accelerations in flow will tend to produce a blunt profile. In turbulent flow, the flow no longer moves in laminae but in irregular unpredictable directions,

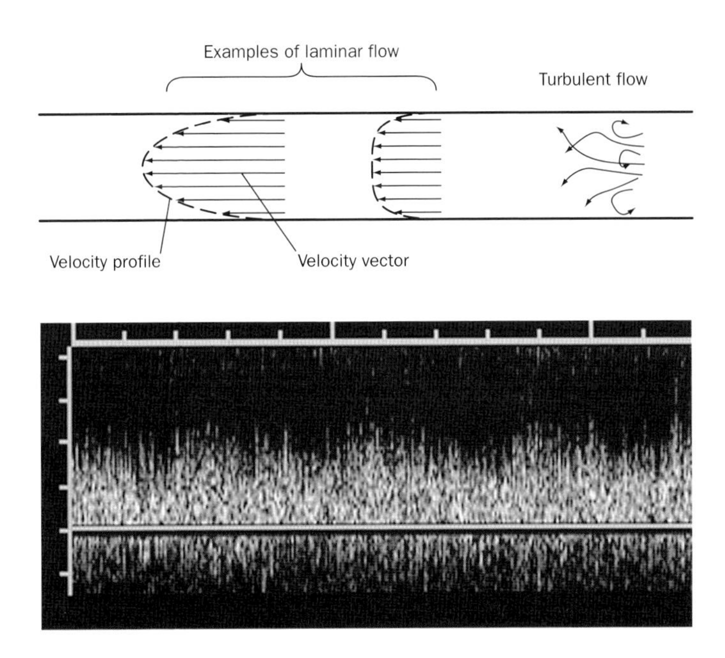

Figure 3.2 Top: flow profiles in laminar (left and center) and turbulent (right) flow in a vessel. Bottom: the sonogram shows the disturbed flow typical in turbulent flow.

including motion across the vessel. Examples of laminar and turbulent flow are shown diagrammatically in Fig. 3.2.

DOPPLER MEASUREMENTS OF BLOOD FLOW

Investigation of fetal and maternal circulation is made using flow waveform analysis, measurement of velocities and measurement of flows. The advantages and disadvantages of each are listed in Table 3.1.

Table 3.1 Advantages and disadvantages of flow waveform analysis, measurement of velocities and measurement of flows

	Advantages	Disadvantages
Flow waveform shape	Does not require beam/vessel angle correction Is reproducible across different ultrasound systems	Does not provide quantitative flow Indices are most useful for measurement of arterial flow; less well proven for venous applications
	Provides qualitative information on the circulation and changes in the circulation Large database of results for fetal and maternal circulation, with proven diagnostic capabilities	

Blood flow velocities	A measure of quantity; increases in velocities in a vessel can imply increase in flow Can be measured reliably if beam/vessel angle correction is made	Beam/vessel angle correction must be correct Mean velocity measurements are subject to instrumentation errors Less data available than for flow waveform analysis
Volume flow measurements	Quantified volume flow	Requires measurement of vessel area/diameter, which is possible in only comparatively large vessels Requires measurement of mean velocity in the spectrum Difficult to get accurate results; very large errors are possible and likely Data collection is at an early stage for fetal/maternal applications

HOW TO DO IT

Flow Waveform Indices – How To Measure Them

Figure 3.1 shows an arterial flow waveform with some of the measurements that are used to analyze flow. The common flow waveform indices use measurements of the outline of the waveform. Shown here are:

- Peak systolic velocity, *S*
- End-diastolic velocity (also the minimum velocity in this waveform), *D*
- Time-averaged maximum velocity, TAMX

These are used in the following common indices:

- Resistance index (RI) = $(S–D)/S$
- S/D ratio = S/D
- Pulsatility index (PI) = $(S–D)/\text{TAMX}$

Resistance index and *S/D* are easy and quick to measure. The PI is more versatile when diastolic flow falls to zero. It can distinguish between waveforms where there is no diastolic flow and those where diastolic flow gradually falls to zero. In both cases RI = 1 and *S/D* is infinity.

Examples of these measurements for uterine arteries showing high and low resistance are shown in Fig. 3.3.

Other measurements of elements of waveform shape include acceleration indices and the presence of a post-systolic notch.

Many manufacturers provide automatic measurement of pulsatility and resistance indices. It is prudent to check index values measured automatically by comparing them against those obtained manually to compare accuracy and consistency.

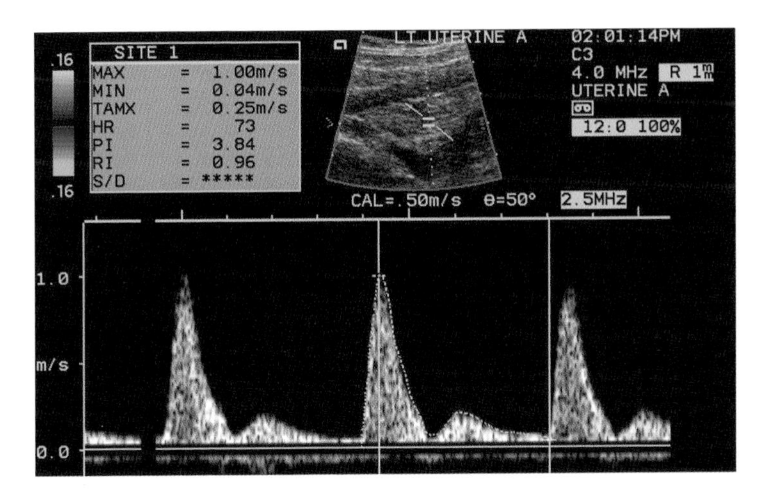

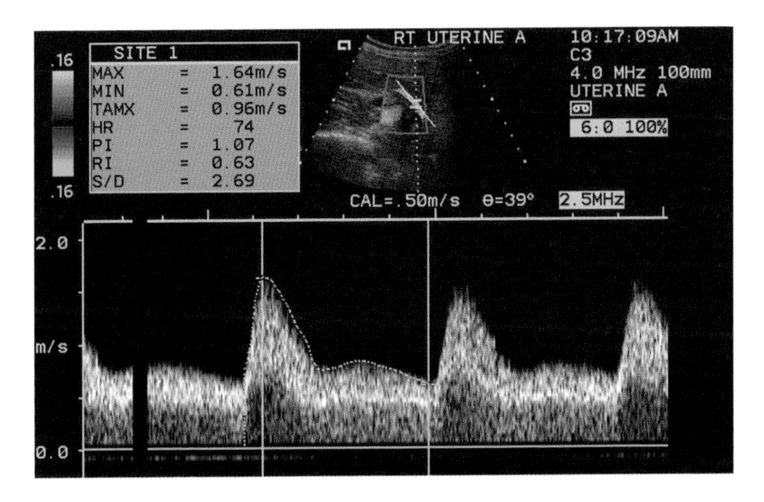

Figure 3.3 Flow waveforms in high (top) and low (bottom) distal resistance flow. The pulsatility and resistance indices show a qualitative measure of the difference in distal resistance.

Measurement of Mean Velocity: Time-averaged Velocity (TAV)

If mean velocity can be measured in a vessel, and the vessel does not change in size, changes in flow can be assessed by changes in mean velocity because blood flow volume = cross-sectional area of a vessel × mean velocity in the vessel.

The time-averaged velocity in Fig. 3.1 is shown approximately by the orange line. An example is shown in Fig. 3.4. Calculation of this is subject to instrumentation errors. Further errors can arise:

- If the vessel is not sampled uniformly across its area
- If a high-wall filter is used (low velocities will be removed and the mean artificially raised) (Fig. 3.5)
- If adjacent vessels are included in the sample volume (Fig. 3.6)

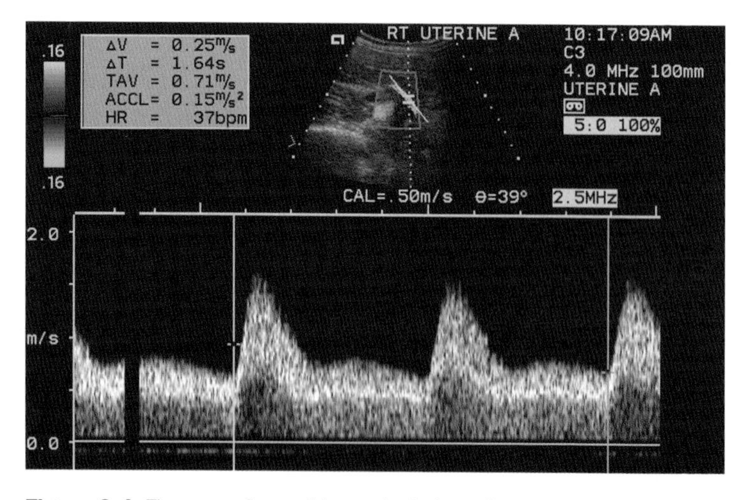

Figure 3.4 Flow waveform with a calculation of time-averaged velocity (TAV). The mean velocity in the sample volume is measured over two cardiac cycles.

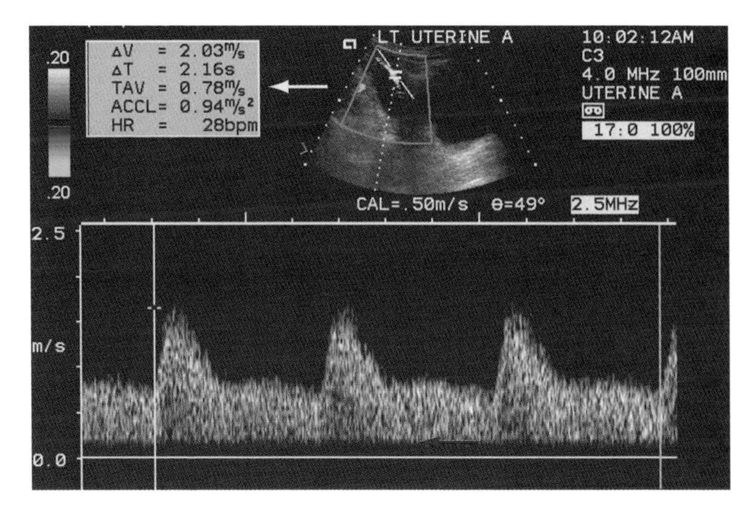

Figure 3.5 High-wall filter (red arrow) removes low velocities and causes the measured time-averaged velocity (TAV) to be elevated (yellow arrow).

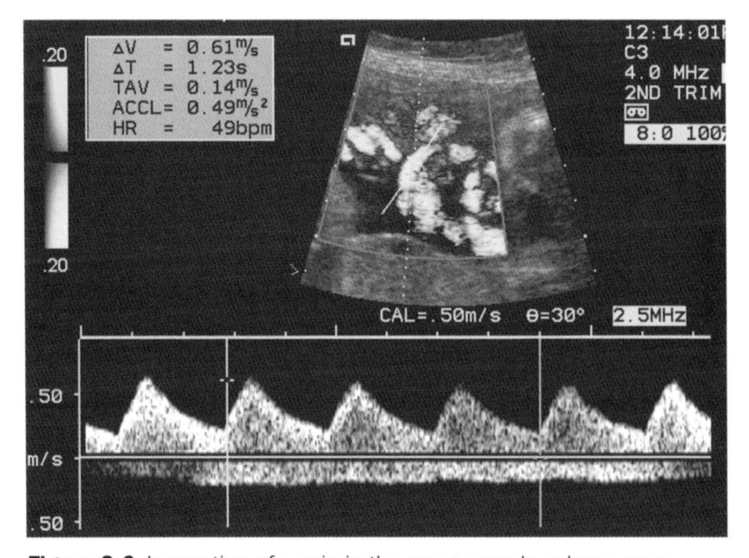

Figure 3.6 Insonation of a vein in the same sample volume as an artery. The venous velocities subtract from the arterial velocities making the time-averaged velocity (TAV) inaccurate.

MEASUREMENT OF VOLUME FLOW

Conventional Doppler volume flow measurements require mean velocity and vessel area (or diameter if the vessel is circular in cross-section). Errors in mean velocity are described above. Errors in diameter can arise from the limited spatial resolution, errors in placing the cursors and errors if the true diameter is not imaged. For example, an error of 0.5 mm in measuring a vessel of diameter 3 mm leads to errors of area over 30%. In combination with velocity measurement errors, volume flow errors of 50% or more are possible.

If volume-flow measurements are being attempted, it is prudent to be aware of possible errors and to conduct tests to ensure results are reproducible.

FURTHER READING

Oates CP (2001) *Cardiovascular Hemodynamics and Doppler Waveforms Explained.* London: Greenwich Medical Media Ltd.

4

ULTRASOUND SAFETY

Ultrasound is a form of energy that can cause thermal and mechanical effects in tissues. To date, there is no evidence that diagnostic ultrasound has been harmful to patients, and patients and ultrasound staff generally perceive it as safe. However, modern scanners operate at higher outputs than earlier machines and, in general, intensities for color-flow imaging and pulsed-wave Doppler are significantly higher than for conventional B-mode. Ultrasound is now so widely used in pregnancy that it is essential for all practitioners to ensure that its use remains safe.

This chapter outlines ultrasound effects and the current regulations and guidelines for safe scanning. It shows how exposure to ultrasound can be kept to within agreed limits while still ensuring good quality diagnostic images.

THERMAL EFFECTS

As ultrasound is absorbed, its energy is converted into heat. The amount of heating depends on variables in both the tissue and the scanner. These include:

- Ultrasound absorption. Heating is highest where there is a high absorption coefficient, particularly in bone, and is low where there is little absorption (e.g. amniotic fluid)

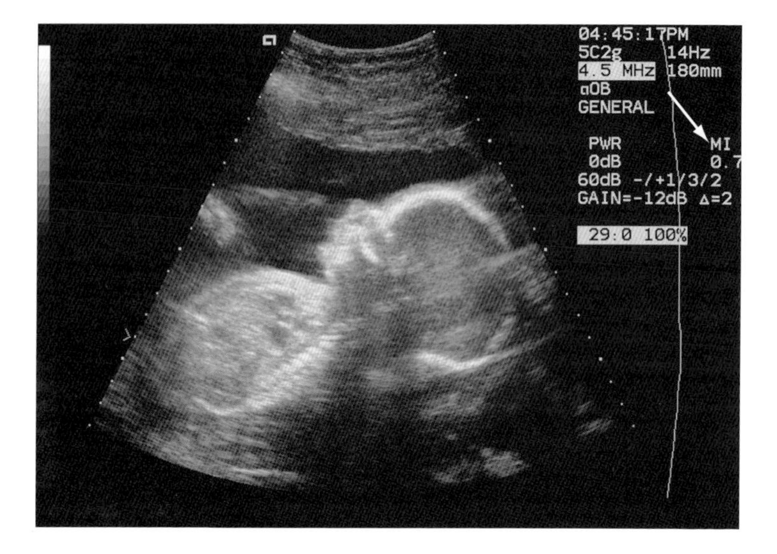

Figure 4.1 The B-mode image of a fetus. The mechanical index (MI) is shown in the data field (arrow).

- Conduction of heat in the tissue, for example into tissue adjacent to bone
- Perfusion
- Ultrasound intensity, which in turn is dependent on the power output and the position of the tissue in the beam profile. The intensity at a point is altered by many of the operator controls, for example power output, mode (B-mode, color-flow imaging or pulsed-wave Doppler), scan depth, focus, zoom and area of color-flow imaging
- Length of time that a volume of tissue is scanned

The transducer face can itself become heated during an examination. Heat is localized to the tissue in contact with the transducer. The transducer face can become warm to the touch if left running exposed to air at high outputs.

High temperatures are known to be a hazard to fetal and embryonic development but the precise sensitivity to heat is incompletely understood. Studies on the effect of heat on tissue are summarized in the references listed in Further Reading. The World Federation of Ultrasound in Medicine and Biology (WFUMB) has stated that ultrasound producing temperature rises of less than 1.5°C may be used without reservation. Temperature rises of greater than 4°C for over 5 min should be considered potentially hazardous. This leaves a range of temperature increase (1.5–4°C), which is within the capability of diagnostic ultrasound equipment to produce and for which there is uncertainty over the biological effects.

MECHANICAL EFFECTS

The passing of a pressure pulse through tissue produces forces that have been shown to produce hemorrhage in animal tissues in the presence of pockets of gas (in the lung and intestines). At high negative pressures, ultrasound can lead to cavitation where there are bubble nuclei. The use of contrast agents increases the risk of cavitation. The precise mechanism for observed hemorrhage has not been identified. The patient group most likely to be at risk from any possible effects is preterm infants. It is not thought that embryos or fetuses are at risk from mechanical effects.

Mechanical effects of ultrasound are sometimes evident as streaming of fluid, for example in amniotic fluid.

OUTPUT REGULATIONS, STANDARDS AND GUIDELINES – WHO DOES WHAT?

Regulations governing the output of diagnostic ultrasound have been largely set by the USA Food and Drug Administration (FDA), although the International Electrotechnical Commission (IEC) is currently in the process of setting internationally agreed standards.

Several national and international societies for ultrasound users have safety committees that offer advice on the safe use of ultrasound. This information is often provided on the Internet (see Table 4.1)

CURRENT STANDARDS

In 1992, the American Institute of Ultrasound in Medicine (AIUM), in conjunction with the National Electrical Manufacturers Association (NEMA) developed the Output Display Standard (ODS) including the Thermal Index and Mechanical Index, which have been incorporated in the FDA's new regulations. At the same time, the maximum intensity limit for obstetric applications was increased nearly eightfold. This has placed the onus on ultrasound users to ensure that exposure is kept within safe limits.

CURRENT REGULATIONS – THE OUTPUT DISPLAY STANDARD

The output display standard is based on two indices: the mechanical index (MI) and the thermal index (TI).

Mechanical Index

The MI (Fig. 4.1) is an estimate of the maximum amplitude of the pressure pulse in tissue. It gives an indication of the relative risk of mechanical effects. The FDA regulations allow MI up to 1.9 to be used for all applications except ophthalmic, which has a maximum of 0.23.

Thermal Index

The TI is the ratio of the power used to that required to cause a maximum temperature increase of 1°C. A TI of 1 indicates a power causing a temperature increase of 1°C. A TI of 2 indicates twice that power (but not necessarily twice the temperature rise).

Because temperature rise is dependent on tissue type and is particularly dependent on the presence of bone, TI is subdivided into three indices:

- TIS – TI for soft tissue
- TIB – TI with bone at/near the focus
- TIC – TI with bone at the surface (e.g. cranial examination)

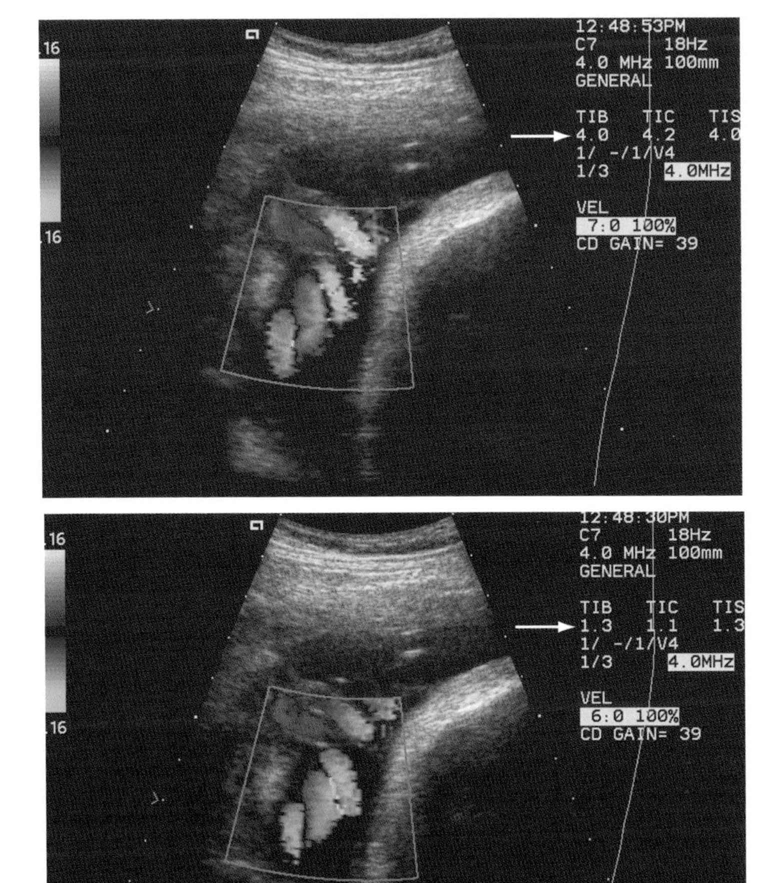

Figure 4.2 Differences in thermal index (TI) with changing output power. With full output power, TIs are high (top). Reduced power lowers TIs (bottom) with no apparent deterioration in the color-flow image. TIB, TI with bone at/near the focus; TIC, TI with bone at the surface; TIS, TI for soft tissue.

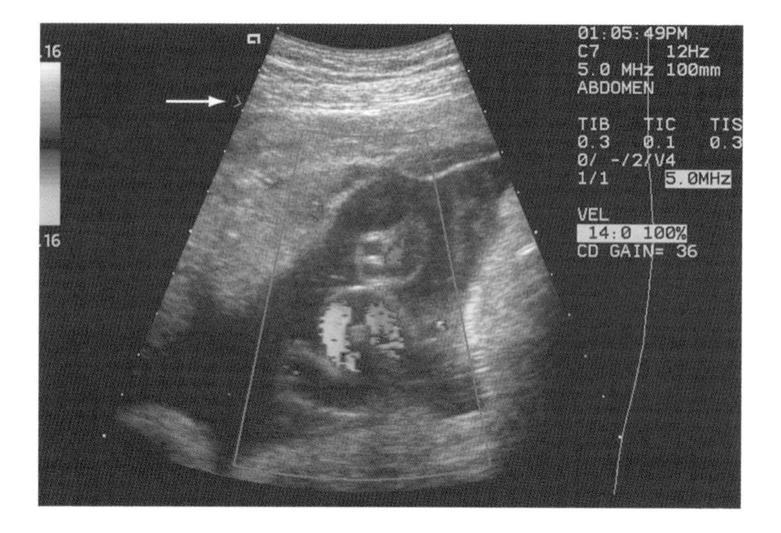

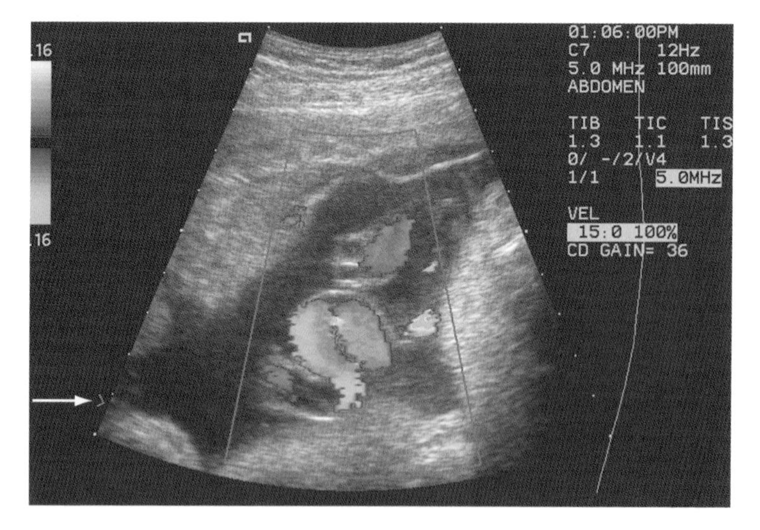

Figure 4.3 Effect of change in focal zone (arrow) on thermal index (TI). No other parameter has been changed in these two images. The TIs are altered by many controls including transmission frequency, color box size, color preprocessing and pulse repetition frequency. TIB, TI with bone at/near the focus; TIC, TI with bone at the surface; TIS, TI for soft tissue.

For fetal scanning, the greatest temperature increase would be expected to occur at bone and TIB would give the 'worst case' conditions. The MI and TI must be displayed if the ultrasound system is capable of exceeding an index of 1.

Thermal indices are very dependent on scanning settings (Figs 4.2 and 4.3), including power output mode (B-mode, color-flow imaging or pulsed-wave Doppler), depth of examination, transmit frequency, color scale (pulse repetition frequency, PRF), size of color box and focus.

Thermal indices are best regarded as a rough guide to the temperature rise that might be produced. Independent studies have suggested that, in some circumstances, temperature rise may be underestimated. The temperature rise itself is dependent on many variables. Guidelines for safe use of ultrasound reflect these uncertainties.

A PRACTICAL APPROACH TO SAFE FETAL SCANNING

No injurious effects have been identified from ultrasound scanning of the fetus. However, changes in power output, increased use of Doppler ultrasound and a change in regulations governing outputs means that operators must take every care to maintain safe practices.

The guidelines for safe scanning practice are:

1. The ALARA (as low as reasonably achievable) principle should be maintained. Power outputs used should be adequate to conduct the examination. Start with a low power and increase it as necessary
2. B-mode generally has the lowest power output and intensity. M-mode, color-flow imaging and pulsed-wave Doppler have higher outputs and can cause more heating at the site of examination. The examination should begin with B-mode and use color-flow imaging and pulsed-wave Doppler only when necessary

Table 4.1 Sources for advice on the safe use of ultrasound

Organization	Abbreviation	Website
American Institute of Ultrasound in Medicine	AIUM	www.aium.org*
British Medical Ultrasound Society	BMUS	www.bmus.org*
Australasian Society for Ultrasound in Medicine	ASUM	www.asum.com.au*
World Federation of Ultrasound in Medicine and Biology	WFUMB	www.wfumb.org
European Federation of Societies for Ultrasound in Medicine and Biology	EFSUMB	www.efsumb.org*

*Website contains guidelines/statements on safety.

Table 4.2 British Medical Ultrasound Society (BMUS) guidelines for maximum recommended times for fetal and embryo scanning

Thermal index (TI)	Maximum exposure time (min)
0.7	60
1.0	30
1.5	15
2.0	4
2.5	1

3 The intensity (and temperature rise) is highly dependent on scanner settings. If the display for the scanner/transducer combination shows TIs and MIs, the indices should be readily visible. Of the thermal indices, TIB is most relevant to heating in the second and third trimester. The operator should be aware of changes to the indices in response to changes in control settings
4 Special care should be taken in febrile patients since ultrasound heating will cause additional heating to the fetus

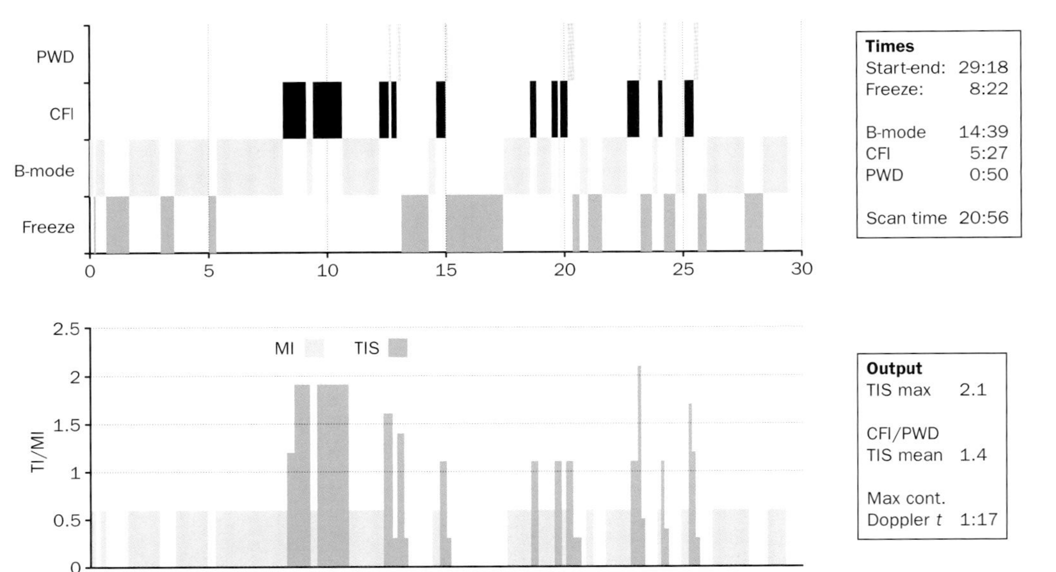

Figure 4.4 Charts of ultrasound use (upper) and mechanical index (MI) and thermal index (TI) levels (lower) during a scan for intrauterine growth retardation (IUGR). The upper chart shows use of B-mode, color-flow imaging (CFI) and pulsed-wave Doppler (PWD) with pauses during which measurements are made. The lower chart shows that exposure reflects this usage, with brief periods of slightly elevated TI during color-flow imaging and pulsed-wave Doppler. TIS, TI for soft tissue. From Deane and Lees (2000).

5 The WFUMB recommends that ultrasound causing a temperature rises of no more than 1.5°C may be used without reservation on thermal grounds
6 TIs exceeding 1.5 should not be used routinely and, if required for specific diagnostic information, should be used for the minimum time necessary. Maximum recommended times for fetal and embryo scanning for different TI levels are given in British Medical Ultrasound Society (BMUS) guidelines (see Table 4.2)
7 Do not scan for longer than is necessary to obtain the diagnostic information

Even in complex scans, these guidelines can be adhered to and good-quality images obtained. Figure 4.4 shows the ultrasound exposure during a scan for intrauterine growth retardation. By starting with B-mode and using color-flow imaging and pulsed-wave Doppler as necessary, exposure to elevated temperatures is kept to a minimum.

FURTHER READING

Barnett SB, Kossoff G (1998) *Safety of Diagnostic Ultrasound*. Carnforth: Parthenon Publishing Group Limited.

Deane C, Lees C (2000) Doppler obstetric ultrasound: a graphical display of output patterns. *Ultrasound Obstet Gynecol* **15,** 418–423.

ter Haar G, Duck FA (2000) *The Safe Use of Ultrasound in Medical Diagnosis*. London: BMUS/BIR.

5

INTEGRATING UTERINE AND FETAL DOPPLER INTO OBSTETRICS

The use of Doppler in perinatal medicine can be divided into two components: uterine artery Doppler (uteroplacental Doppler) and fetal arterial and venous Doppler.

UTERINE ARTERY DOPPLER

Uterine artery Doppler is usually performed as a screening test in a population of pregnant women. This might include all women booking into a particular delivery unit, or those with hypertension, poor pregnancy history or other indication for screening. Screening for high resistance and/or early diagnostic 'notches' allows 'high-risk' women to be identified and appropriate follow-up arrangements to be made.

Because many of the women at risk of the complications of impaired placentation are in their first pregnancy, often no other risk factors are present to alert a clinician to their level of risk.

The complications of impaired placentation are:

- Pre-eclampsia
- Growth restriction
- Placental abruption
- Intrauterine fetal death

Before a uterine Doppler examination is performed, the following demographic and clinical details will help interpret the findings:

- Parity
- Past obstetric history (with particular reference to the complications of impaired placentation)
- Is there a change of partner for this pregnancy?
- Gestational age
- Smoking status
- Ethnicity

Note that there is an association between abnormal uteroplacental Doppler and the later onset of growth restriction and/or fetal growth restriction (Fig. 5.1).

FETAL ARTERIAL AND VENOUS DOPPLER

Fetal Dopplers are usually used in a different context from uterine artery Doppler. Whereas uterine artery Dopplers are usually used for screening, fetal Dopplers are used as an adjunct to diagnosing the severity of fetal compromise in potentially hypoxic conditions. The fetal vessels that may commonly be examined include:

- Umbilical artery
- Umbilical vein
- Middle cerebral artery
- Thoracic aorta
- Ductus venosus

Less commonly, and only in specific indications, the vessels examined include:

- Renal arteries
- Coronary arteries
- Splenic artery

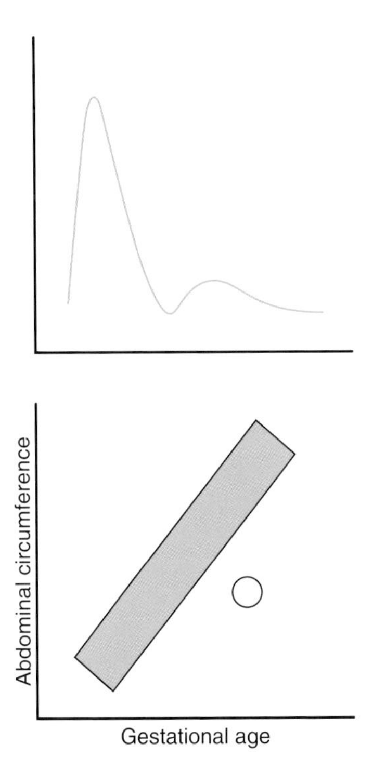

Figure 5.1 Schematic representation of an abnormal uterine artery Doppler waveform (top) with the later onset of fetal growth restriction (bottom).

- Adrenal artery
- Hepatic veins
- Inferior vena cava

Fetal Dopplers are often performed serially in a fetus that is thought to be at 'high risk', and hence requiring close obstetric surveillance. The reasons for this might include growth restriction, reduced amniotic fluid or movements, or maternal hypertension or diabetes.

Before a fetal Doppler examination is performed, it is useful to establish the indication for this Doppler examination and how the results will be used clinically. The management of a mother and fetus depends upon piecing together the whole pattern of movements, fetal growth, and maternal condition to which the added information of Doppler is often very valuable. It is therefore important not to determine obstetric management purely on the basis of Doppler measurements.

The following information is essential in helping to interpret fetal Dopplers:

- Fetal movements
- Amniotic fluid index
- Growth pattern
- Gestation with respect to fetal viability
- Cardiotocograph (preferably with computer analysis of short-term variation)
- Pregnancy history

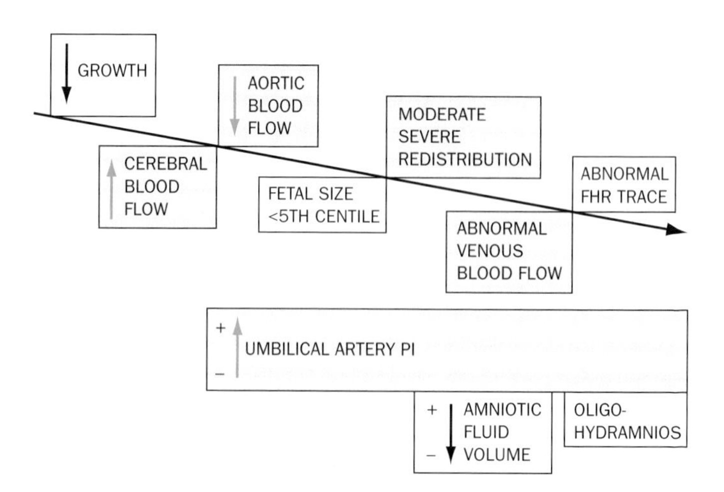

Figure 5.2 The sequence of changes in growth, amniotic fluid and Doppler parameters in uteroplacental insufficiency.

Amniotic fluid : Normal
AF index : 19.5
Placenta : High anterior, Normal
Presentation : Breech

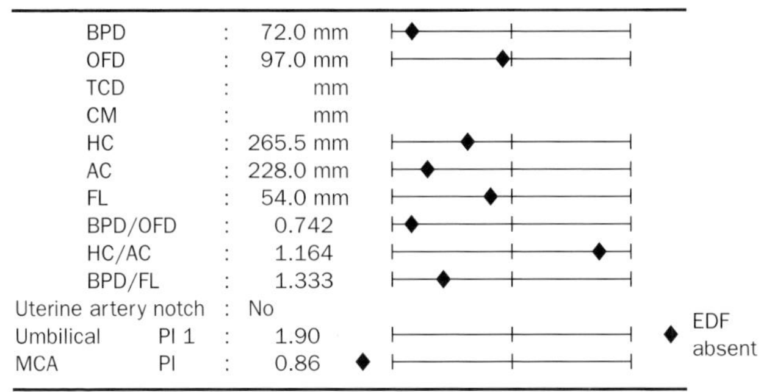

BPD		:	72.0 mm
OFD		:	97.0 mm
TCD		:	mm
CM		:	mm
HC		:	265.5 mm
AC		:	228.0 mm
FL		:	54.0 mm
BPD/OFD		:	0.742
HC/AC		:	1.164
BPD/FL		:	1.333
Uterine artery notch		:	No
Umbilical	PI 1	:	1.90
MCA	PI	:	0.86

Diagnosis : None
Fetal activity : Reduced
Estimated fetal weight : 1150g
Decision : Referred

Figure 5.3 A report generated on dedicated fetal medicine reporting software showing all relevant parameters, including growth, estimated fetal weight, umbilical and middle cerebral pulsatility index, movements and amniotic fluid. This particular case was of rapid-onset fetal asphyxia.

The exact timing of abnormalities of amniotic fluid, growth and Dopplers is variable but can be generalized (see Fig. 5.2). Parameters including growth, amniotic fluid, fetal movements and arterial Dopplers are shown in a typical software-generated report in Fig. 5.3.

6

THE UTERINE ARTERY

The uterine artery is a branch of the internal iliac artery close to the bifurcation of the common iliac artery (Fig. 6.1). As the uterine artery ascends within the uterus, it branches extensively into arcuate and radial vessels, which eventually terminate as spiral arteries. The spiral arteries form the interface with the placenta, in that blood is ejected from the spiral arteries at high velocity and perfuses the intracotyledonary space. The uterine artery is unique among vessels in that it has a remarkable ability to increase its capacity. The blood flow through the non-pregnant uterine artery is roughly 40 mL/min each side, but this increases up to tenfold, to 400 mL/min, by late pregnancy.

Using color-flow imaging, it is possible to place the pulse Doppler gate over a specific part of a particular vessel with accuracy. When visualized transabdominally in the second and third trimester of pregnancy, the uterine artery is usually insonated over its apparent 'crossover', the external iliac artery. This gives a reproducible Doppler landmark for repeat pulse-wave Doppler measurements to be made. There is usually one uterine artery on each side, entering the uterus at the level of the internal cervical os, but it may branch at or before the 'crossover' (Fig. 6.2). If the uterine artery is visualized transvaginally, it is normally insonated at the level of the internal os.

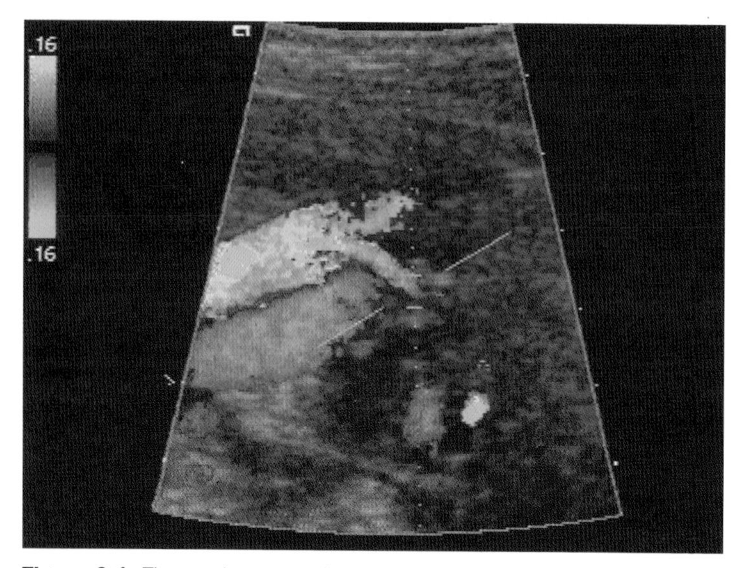

Figure 6.1 The uterine artery (shown in red) at the 'crossover' with the external iliac artery (shown in orange/green).

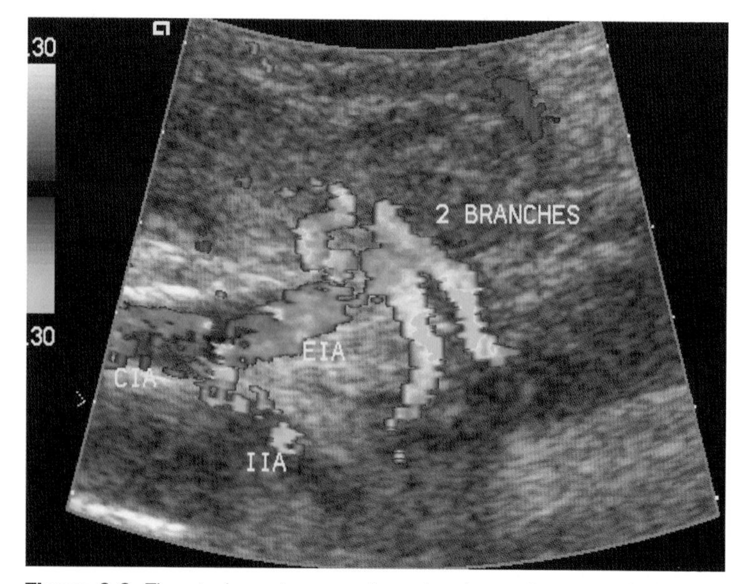

Figure 6.2 The uterine artery may branch prior to the apparent 'crossover' with the external iliac artery.

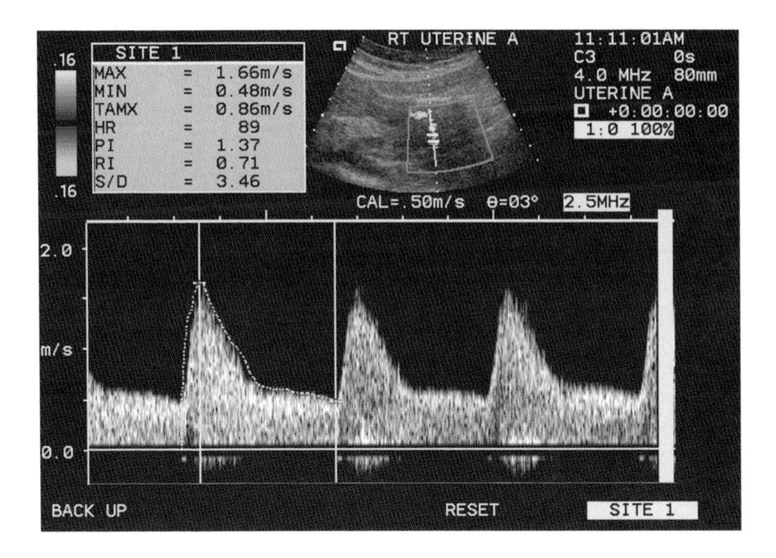

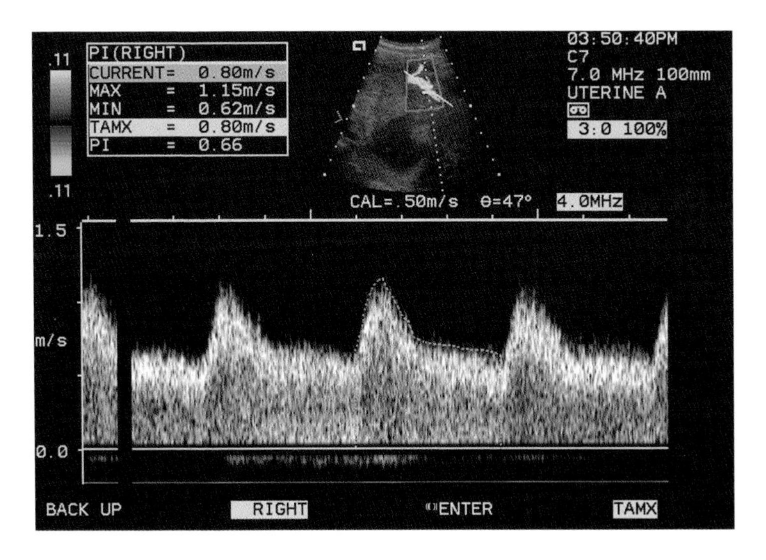

Figure 6.3 Normal uterine artery Doppler waveforms at 23 weeks. In both the pulsatility index (PI) is < 1.45 (95th percentile cut-off at 22–24 weeks).

At this point, pulsed-wave Doppler is applied and once three consecutive consistent waveforms have been obtained, the picture is frozen and indices obtained.

Three abnormalities of uterine artery flow are described:

- High mean resistance (average of left and right uterine arteries) > 95th percentile for resistance index (RI) or pulsatility index (PI)
- Unilateral uterine artery notch
- Bilateral uterine artery notches

Uterine artery waveforms may exhibit a low resistance pattern (Fig. 6.3); these waveforms would be a reassuring finding at 20–24 weeks' gestation.

It is important to ensure that the vessel under investigation is the uterine artery, and not an arcuate branch, as this may lead to an apparent falsely low resistance. This is because the further 'downstream' the uterine artery is insonated, to arcuate, radial, and eventually spiral vessels, the lower the resistance appears.

Uterine artery screening is most commonly carried out at 20–24 weeks' gestation. At this stage, the 'second wave' of trophoblast invasion is complete and those women with abnormal waveforms, either high resistance or bilateral uterine artery notches, are at high risk of developing the complications of impaired placentation. These complications are pre-eclampsia, fetal growth restriction, intrauterine death or placental abruption. Doppler waveforms such as those demonstrated in Fig. 6.4 suggest that close monitoring of the pregnancy is indicated.

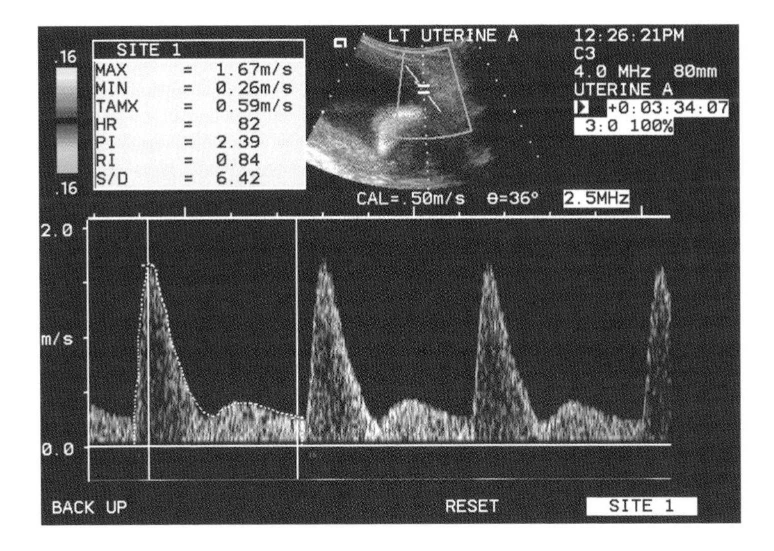

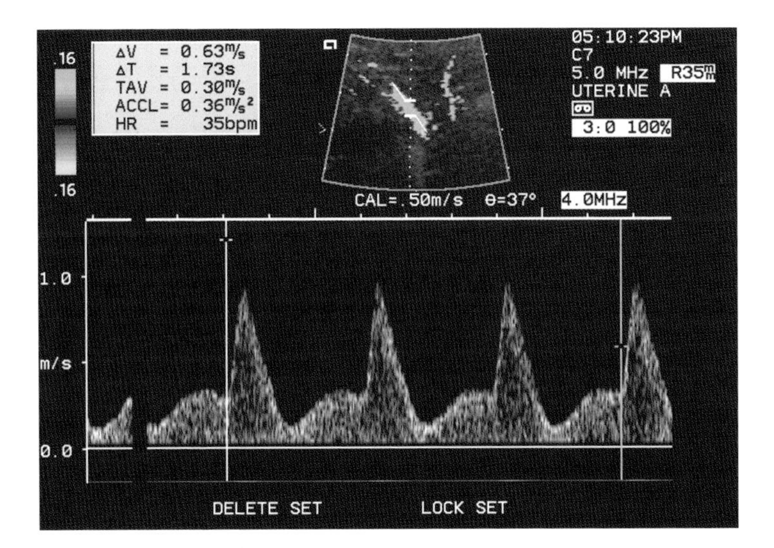

Figure 6.4 Abnormal uterine artery waveforms. Both have notches and high resistance patterns; the top one shows an exceptionally high pulsatility index (PI) (greater than 2.00).

KEY POINTS

- Uterine artery notches are present in almost all women at conception, and most in early pregnancy. They should disappear by 24 weeks; at this stage of gestation in most populations fewer than 5% of women still have bilateral uterine artery notches. Notches do not reappear later in gestation. If notches were present at 24 weeks but disappear thereafter, the risk of pre-eclampsia, intrauterine growth retardation (IUGR) and related complications remains.
- Unilateral uterine artery notches are quite common up to 24 weeks. They confer a slightly higher risk of adverse outcome related to pre-eclampsia and IUGR, but do not on their own constitute a sufficiently high-risk group to justify frequent monitoring unless the mean resistance is > 95th percentile.
- High uterine artery resistance in the absence of notches also selects a high-risk group of women. Because uterine artery resistance (RI or PI) is a continuous measure, the level of risk can be determined by applying this measurement to a chart giving the likelihood of adverse outcome (Appendix B).

FURTHER READING

Bower S, Bewley S, Campbell S (1993) Improved prediction of preeclampsia by two-stage screening of uterine arteries using the early diastolic notch and color Doppler imaging. *Obstet Gynecol* **82**(1), 78–83.

Lees C (2000) Uterine artery Doppler: time to establish the ground rules. Ultrasound. *Obstet Gynecol* **16**(7), 607–9.

Lees C, Parra M, Missfelder-Lobos H, Morgans A, Fletcher O, Nicolaides KH (2001) Individualized risk assessment for adverse pregnancy outcome by uterine artery Doppler at 23 weeks. *Obstet Gynecol* **98**(3), 369–73.

7

FETAL ARTERIAL AND VENOUS DOPPLER

THE UMBILICAL ARTERY WAVEFORM

Umbilical artery Doppler is not synonymous with fetal Doppler. The umbilical artery waveform represents placental, not fetal, vascular resistance. It should therefore be regarded primarily as an indicator of resistance in the feto-placental vascular bed.

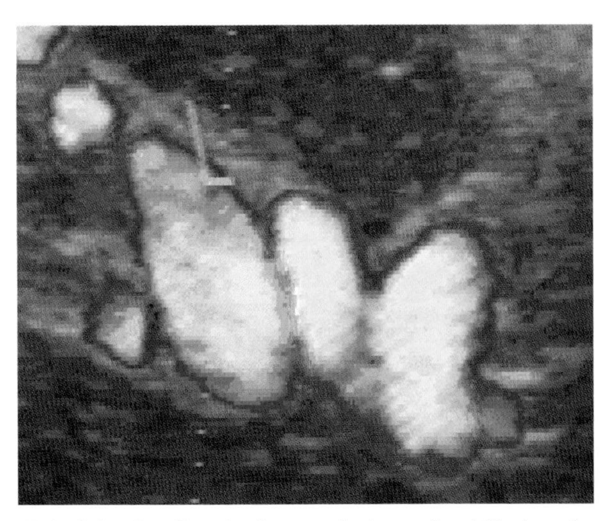

Figure 7.1 Color-flow Doppler image of a loop of umbilical cord showing the typical two arteries and one vein, with blood flowing in opposite directions.

Umbilical artery waveforms can be obtained from either artery using continuous-wave or color-flow imaging equipment. Figure 7.1 shows two arteries (yellow) and the larger umbilical vein (blue). Waveforms are usually obtained from a free loop of umbilical cord, in most cases near the placental insertion where movement artifact is less. The angle should ideally be less than 60° (Fig. 7.2). There is no consistent significant difference in the shape of the waveform, depending upon where the cord is insonated, neither is it common for there to be a difference in waveform between the two arteries.

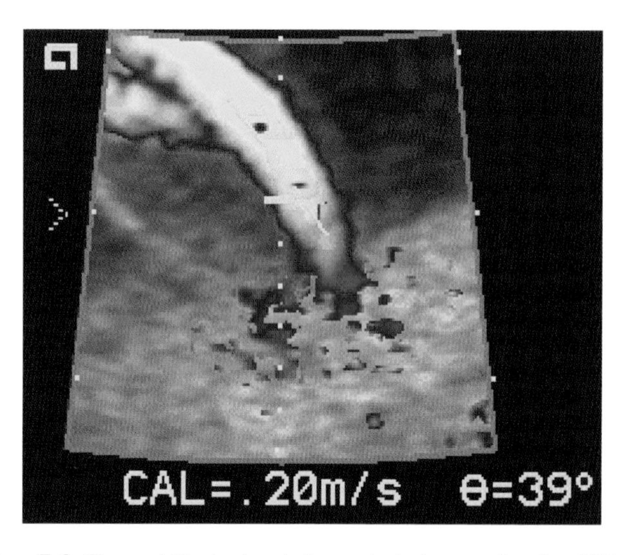

Figure 7.2 The umbilical artery is insonated at an angle of < 60°.

Three major abnormalities of umbilical artery flow are described:

- Raised resistance (pulsatility index (PI) or resistance index (RI) >95th percentile)
- Absent end-diastolic flow (EDF)
- Reversed EDF

From 16 weeks onwards, the umbilical artery waveform should show positive EDF (Fig. 7.3). Reduction in EDF, a rise in PI,

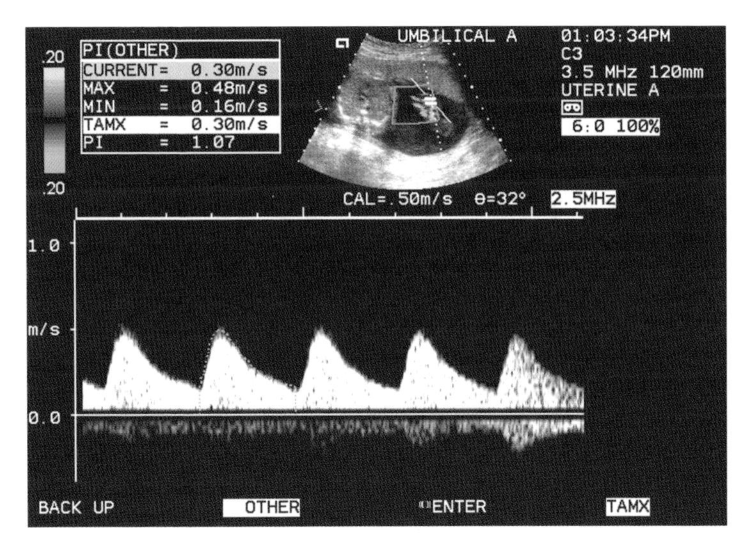

Figure 7.3 Normal umbilical artery Doppler with positive end-diastolic flow (EDF).

absent EDF (Fig. 7.4), and reversed EDF (Fig. 7.5) represent a chronological continuum of increasing feto-placental resistance. At 24–30 weeks, a fetus may have absent EDF in the umbilical artery for several weeks, or even reversed EDF for several days before delivery is necessary. This is why, at early gestation, absent or reversed EDF in the umbilical artery should not, without corroborating evidence from other fetal Doppler measurements, be the sole indication for delivery. At 30–34 weeks, delivery decisions in a growth-restricted baby may be made on the basis of amniotic fluid index, movements, cardiotocograph (CTG) and umbilical artery Doppler. After 34 weeks, abnormal umbilical artery Doppler (absent or reversed EDF) is unusual and almost always suggests severe feto-placental pathology warranting delivery.

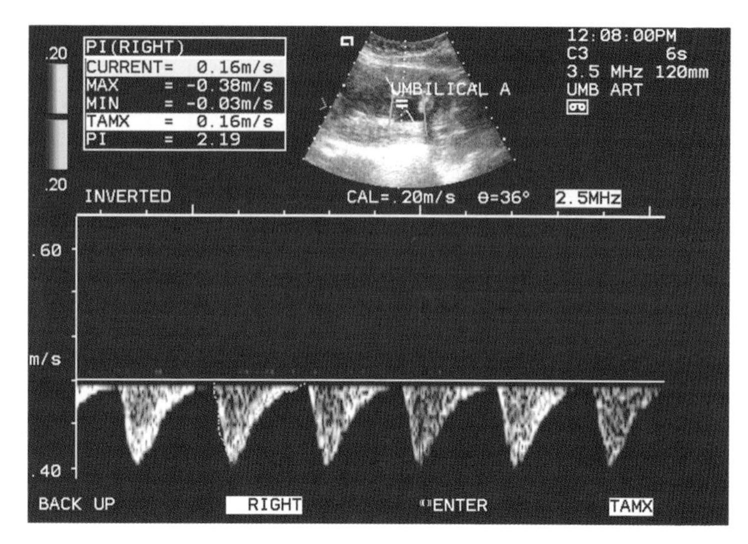

Figure 7.4 Abnormal umbilical artery Doppler with absent end-diastolic flow.

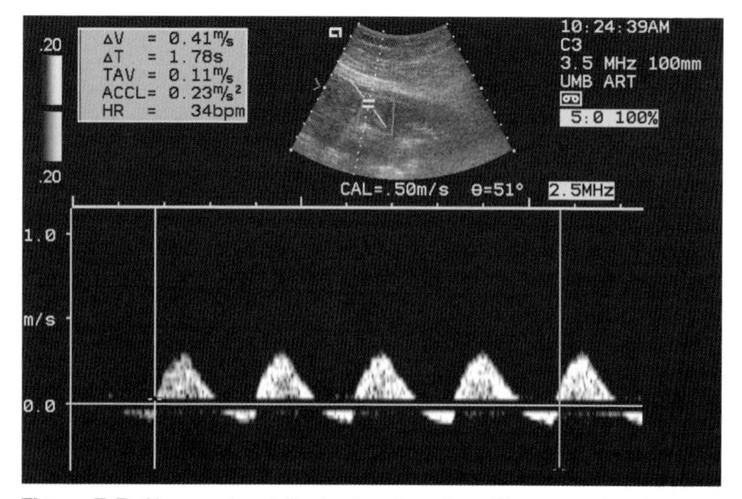

Figure 7.5 Abnormal umbilical artery Doppler with reversed end-diastolic flow.

Key Points

- Umbilical artery Doppler is not synonymous with fetal Doppler.
- Umbilical artery Doppler gives an indication about feto-placental vascular resistance. This does not necessarily correlate Doppler findings of the fetal circulation.
- Absent or reversed umbilical artery end-diastolic flow is not a diagnosis or the basis on which delivery should be decided. It suggests more detailed investigation in units where fetal Doppler is available or close observation and investigation using a cardiotocograph in units where it is not.

THE MIDDLE CEREBRAL ARTERY

The fetal head is visualized in the biparietal diameter section, and the probe tilted to allow visualization of the greater wing of the sphenoid bone. The course of the middle cerebral artery (MCA)

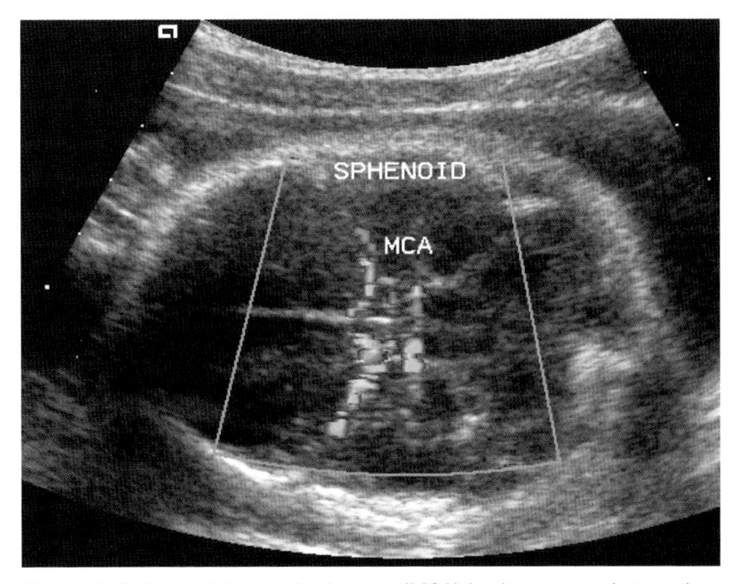

Figure 7.6 The middle cerebral artery (MCA) is shown coursing up the wing of the sphenoid bone, with the fetal head in the transverse position.

follows the wing of the sphenoid bone, allowing it to be seen easily on color-flow wave Doppler (Fig. 7.6). The anterior vessel is insonated with pulsed Doppler in the segment nearest the circle of Willis. This is known as the M1 segment of the MCA (Fig. 7.7). Care should be taken to avoid pressure with the transducer on the fetal head, which has been shown to increase the MCA PI transiently. The fetal head, especially if lying in cephalic presentation, is usually in the transverse plane, allowing the cerebral artery to be visualized easily.

The normal MCA waveform from 22 to 28 weeks shows little or no EDF (Fig. 7.8). It is not uncommon to see a little reverse flow even in a healthy fetus (Fig. 7.9). From 28 to 34 weeks, a little EDF is often seen, but this is normal. After 34 weeks, 'physiological redistribution' (i.e. a reduction in MCA resistance) may occur

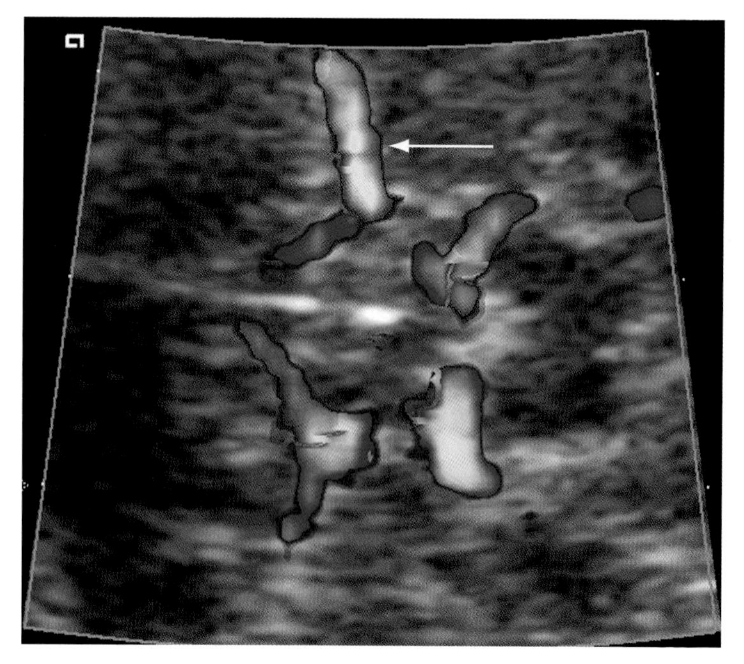

Figure 7.7 The circle of Willis showing middle and posterior cerebral artery branches. Arrow shows M1 segment of the MCA.

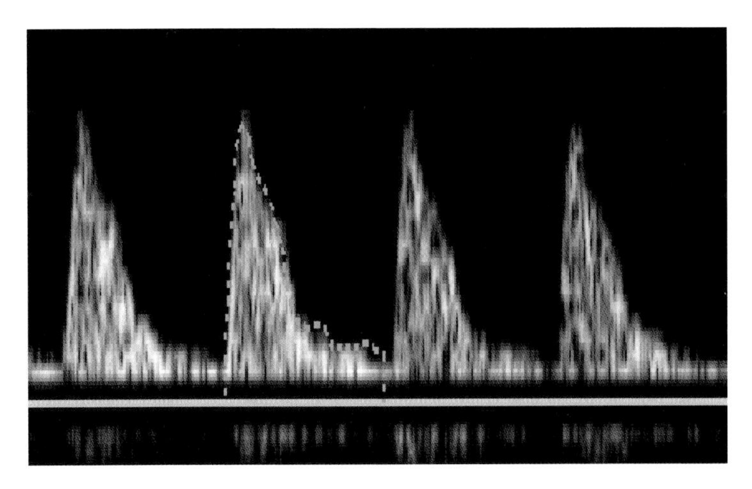

Figure 7.8 Normal middle cerebral artery waveform showing a small 'trickle' of diastolic flow.

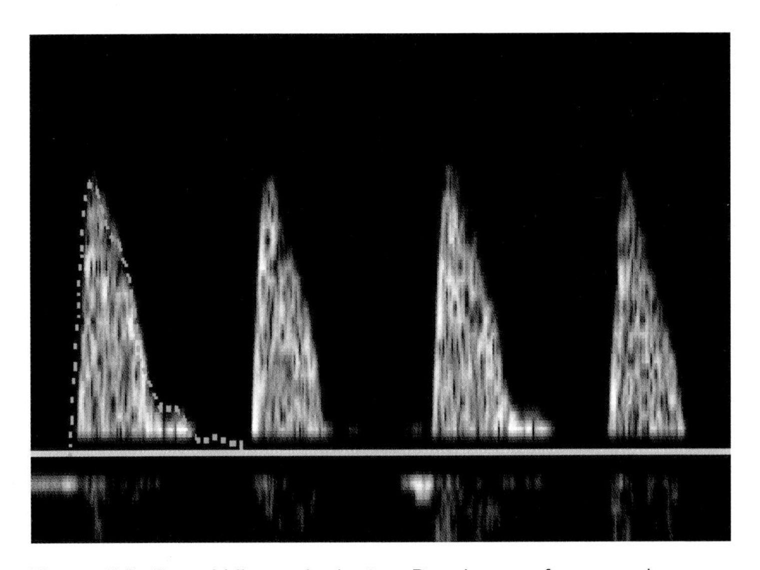

Figure 7.9 The middle cerebral artery Doppler waveform may, in normal circumstances, show absent or even a slight reversal in end-diastolic flow.

owing to changes in flow through the heart, leading to relatively deoxygenated blood being shunted to the cerebral circulation.

In hypoxia, there is a progressive reduction in resistance in the MCA (Fig. 7.10). In conditions of severe hypoxia leading to fetal acidemia (fetal decompensation), the fetal MCA PI may show a paradoxical increase in resistance for a short while (usually 24–48 h) before irreversible fetal heart rate changes or fetal death occur.

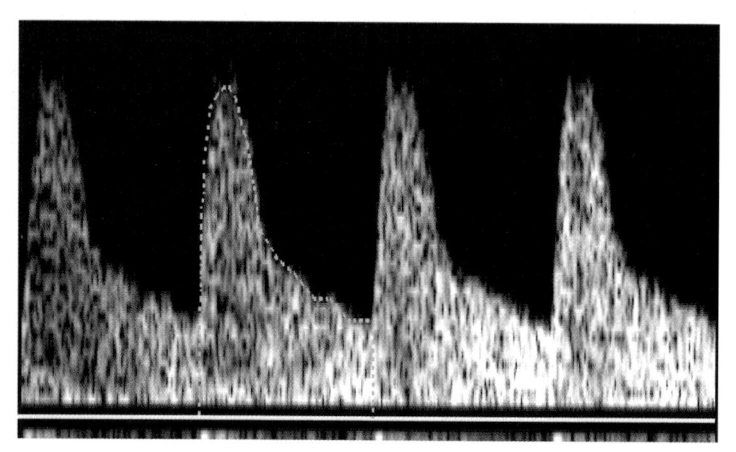

Figure 7.10 Extensive end-diastolic flow in the middle cerebral artery suggesting cerebral redistribution (brain-sparing effect).

THE THORACIC AORTA

The thoracic aorta is the least important vessel to visualize in the investigation of fetal condition. Little extra information can be gained that has not already been ascertained from the umbilical and middle cerebral arteries, and the vessel may be technically difficult to image.

A longitudinal sagittal view of the fetus should be obtained (Fig. 7.11), and the thoracic (supra-diaphragmatic) segment of the aorta viewed using color-flow imaging (Fig. 7.12). This position should be far enough away from the heart for the waveform to be unaffected by interference from cardiac vessels, but should be

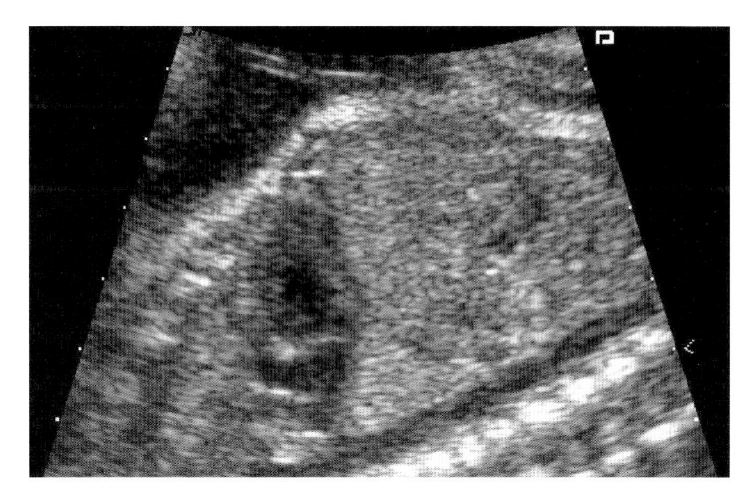

Figure 7.11 The fetal chest is seen in sagittal section, showing the supra-diaphragmatic aorta.

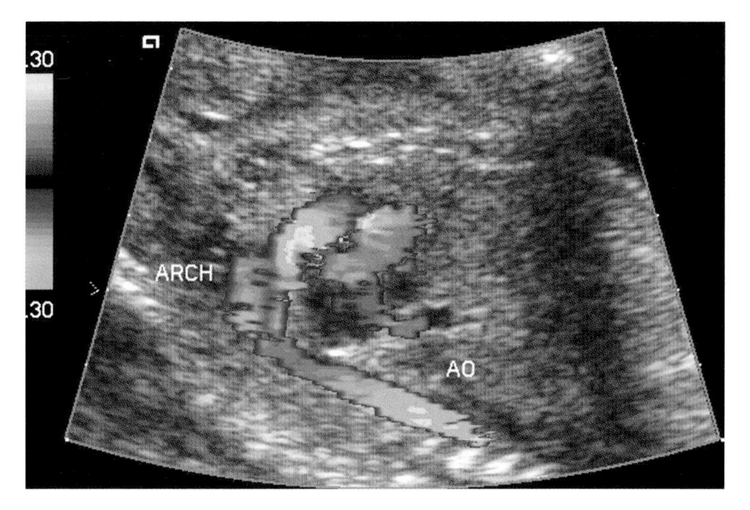

Figure 7.12 Color-flow imaging is applied, showing the arch and thoracic aorta.

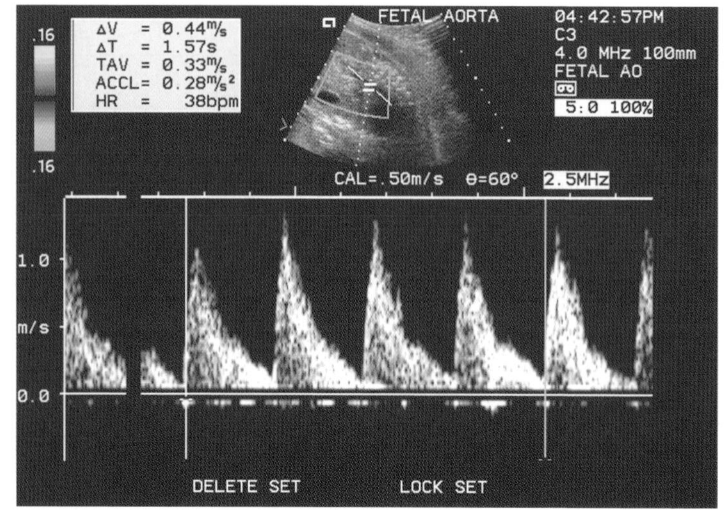

(a)

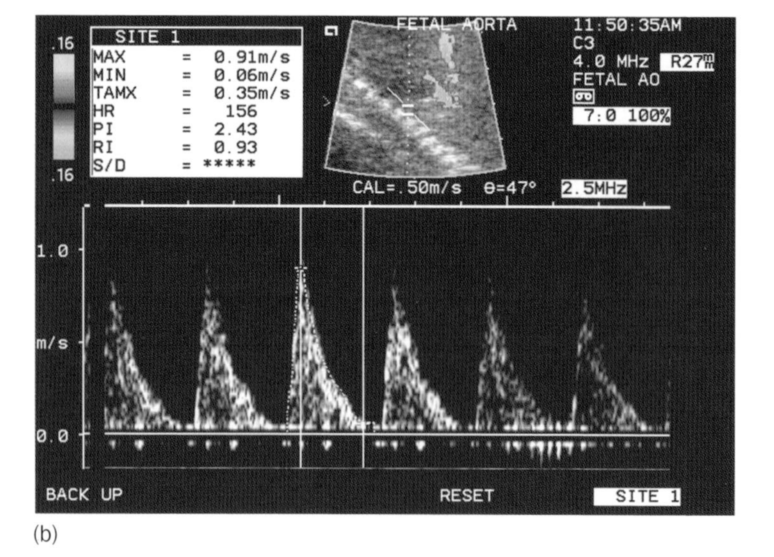

(b)

Figure 7.13 Thoracic aorta waveforms showing normal (a), reduced (b), absent (c) and reversed (d) end-diastolic flow.

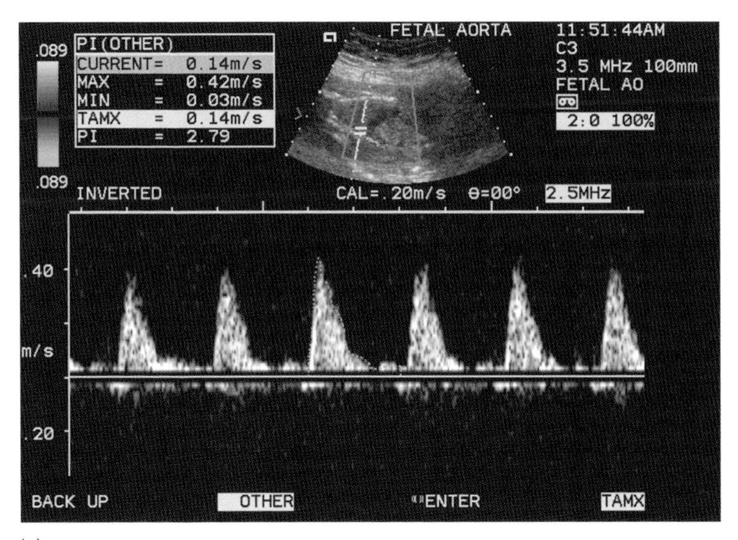
.089
PI(OTHER)
CURRENT= 0.14m/s
MAX = 0.42m/s
MIN = 0.03m/s
TAMX = 0.14m/s
PI = 2.79
FETAL AORTA
11:51:44AM
C3
3.5 MHz 100mm
FETAL AO
2:0 100%
.089
INVERTED
CAL=.20m/s θ=00°
2.5MHz
.40
m/s
.20
BACK UP
OTHER
ENTER
TAMX

(c)

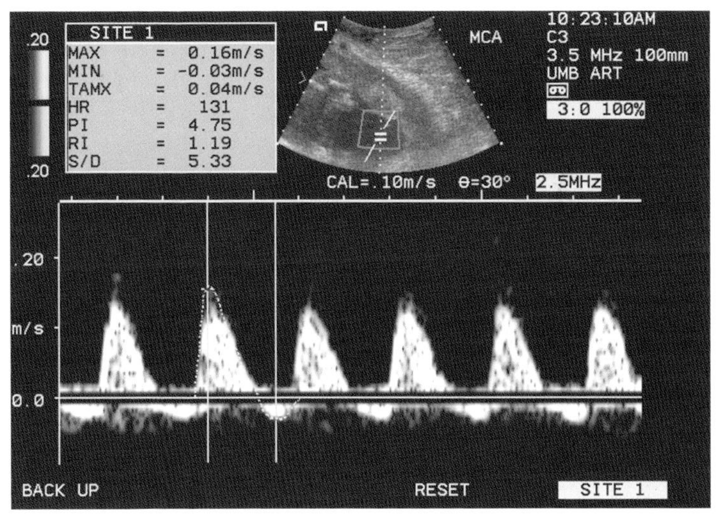
.20
SITE 1
MAX = 0.16m/s
MIN = -0.03m/s
TAMX = 0.04m/s
HR = 131
PI = 4.75
RI = 1.19
S/D = 5.33
MCA
10:23:10AM
C3
3.5 MHz 100mm
UMB ART
3:0 100%
.20
CAL=.10m/s θ=30°
2.5MHz
.20
m/s
0.0
BACK UP
RESET
SITE 1

(d)

above the diaphragm. With an angle of less than 60°, pulsed-wave Doppler is applied to obtain a consistent series of flow waveform velocities (FVWs) without fetal breathing movements being present. Fetal breathing movements make the thoracic aorta waveform uninterpretable; the measurement should therefore be performed again after a pause of 10–20 min.

It is normal for there to be EDF from approximately 20 weeks onwards (Fig. 7.13a). Progressive fetal hypoxia leads to reduced, absent and reversed EDF (Fig. 7.13b–d).

Key Point

- Fetal Dopplers may become abnormal even in normally growing babies. This may occur with rapid onset pre-eclampsia or poorly controlled diabetes (the latter usually with maternal metabolic acidosis).

FETAL VENOUS DOPPLERS

Umbilical Vein

The umbilical vein is often overlooked because of its more frequently investigated neighbor, the umbilical artery. In severe fetal compromise or heart failure, the umbilical vein can give important information especially if for technical reasons the fetal ductus venosus cannot be visualized.

The normal umbilical venous waveform, from the late second trimester onwards, exhibits a low-velocity continuous flow. Using pulsed-wave Doppler, it is often obtained superimposed on an umbilical artery waveform. Beware of confusing umbilical vein pulsations with the common physiological undulations associated with fetal breathing; the latter are low amplitude and irregular and of no pathological significance.

Ductus Venosus

The ductus venosus is the short, narrow connection between the umbilical vein and the heart (Figs 7.14 and 7.15). Oxygenated

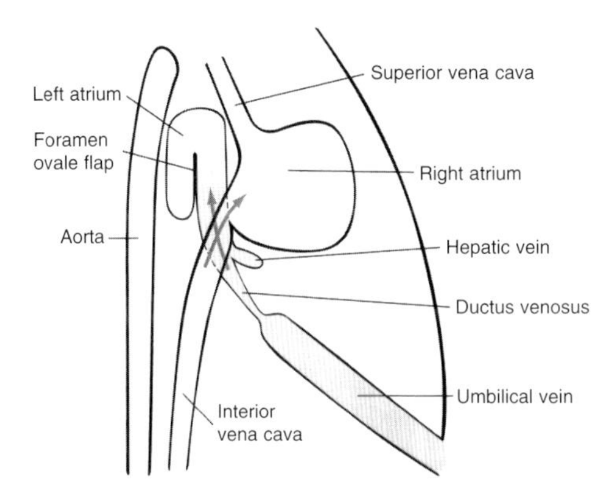

Figure 7.14 The anatomy of the ductus venosus.

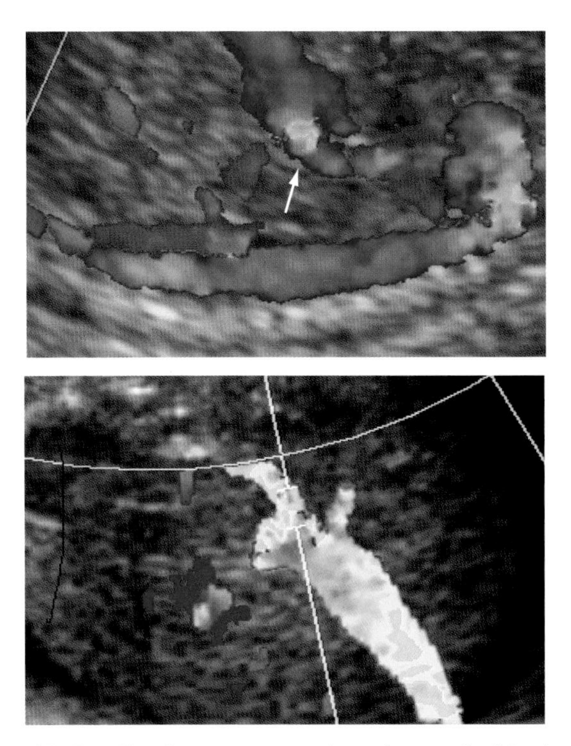

Figure 7.15 Top: The ductus venosus shown in a sagittal fetal section, with a color change, suggesting higher velocities passing through the 'funnel' of the ductus. Bottom: The ductus venosus shown in a transverse fetal section, in continuity with the umbilical vein as it gives off hepatic branches.

blood is directed from the umbilical vein into the fetal circulation towards the foramen ovale. The blood flow in the ductus venosus therefore reflects the pressure gradient between these two structures. It is not to be confused with the ductus arteriosus, which carries blood bypassing the fetal lungs from the right ventricle to the aorta.

The ductus venosus waveform is clearly distinguishable from that of the inferior vena cava and hepatic vein. These vessels are very close to each other, so it is possible, if the gate width is set too large, to obtain a composite waveform containing several vessels, which will lead to inaccurate interpretation. It is important to note that the sound of the ductus venosus Doppler waveform is distinctly different from that of other neighboring veins, and that it is possible, with some experience, to recognize the high-pitch continuous 'hissing' sound of the ductus. This is quite different from the inferior vena cava and hepatic veins. The typical ductus venosus waveform, with 's', 'd' and 'a' waves is shown in Fig. 7.16.

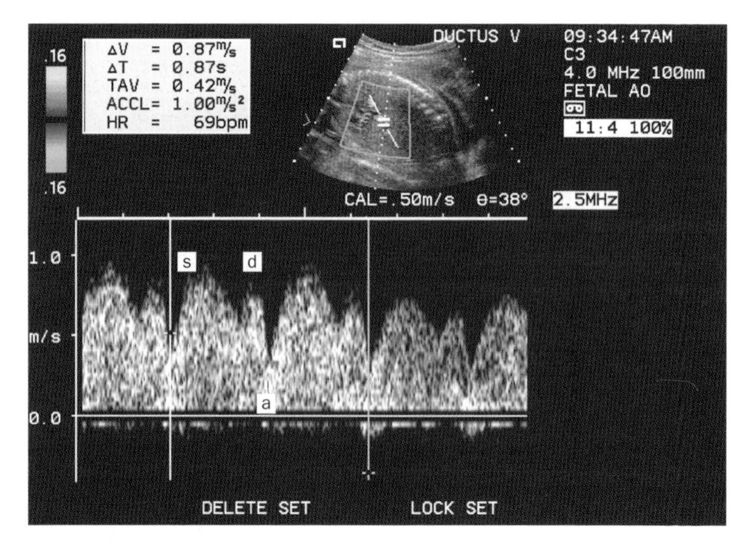

Figure 7.16 A normal ductus venosus waveform with 's', 'd' and 'a' waves shown.

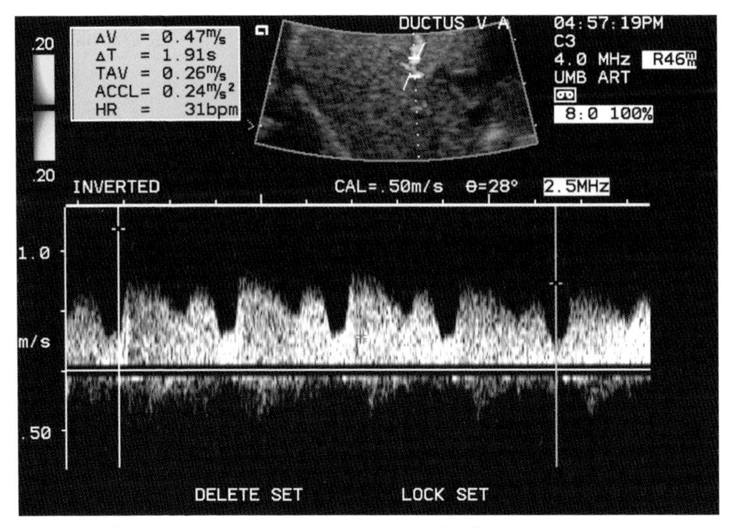

Figure 7.17(a) Ductus venous exaggerated 'a' wave.

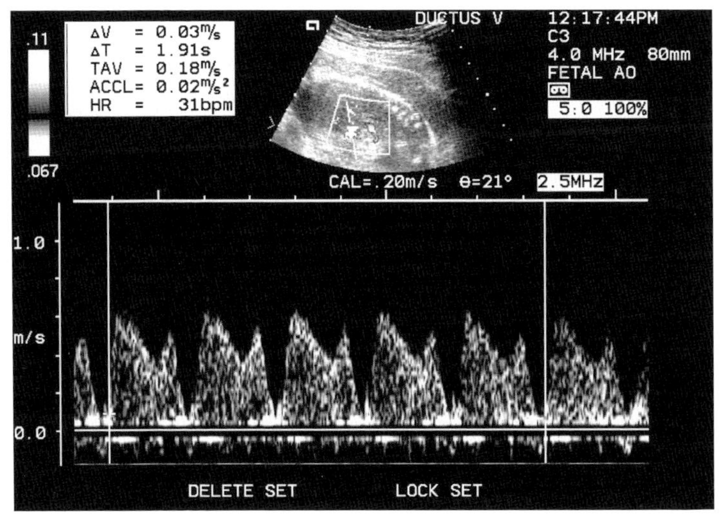

Figure 7.17(b) Ductus venous with 'a' wave reaching the baseline.

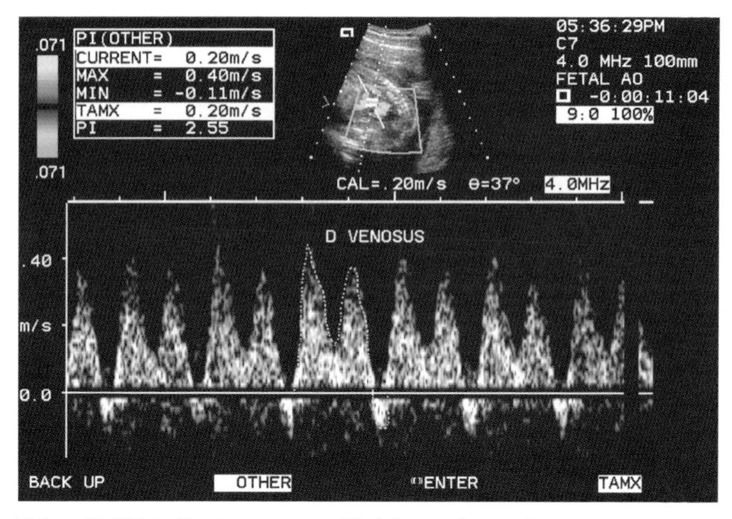

Figure 7.17(c) Ductus venous with 'a' wave becoming reversed.

Ductus venosus abnormalities can be categorized as:

- Raised ductus resistance (pulsatility index (venous), PIV) > 95th percentile) (Fig. 7.17a)
- Exaggerated 'a' wave approaching the baseline (Fig. 7.17b)
- Reversed 'a' wave ('a' wave beneath the baseline) (Fig. 7.17c)

A reversed 'a' wave is an ominous sign and suggests fetal decompensation. This may occur in the recipient in twin-to-twin transfusion syndrome and, in the context of uteroplacental insufficiency, severe hypoxia/acidemia. It may also occur in end-stage fetal anemia or viral myocarditis.

FURTHER READING

Baschat AA, Gembruch U, Reiss I, Gortner L, Weiner CP, Harman CR (2000) Relationship between arterial and venous Doppler and perinatal outcome in fetal growth restriction. *Ultrasound Obstet Gynecol* **16**(5), 407–13.

Harrington KF (2000) Making best and appropriate use of fetal biophysical and Doppler ultrasound data in the management of the growth restricted fetus. *Ultrasound Obstet Gynecol* **16**(5), 399–401.

Harrington K, Thompson MO, Carpenter RG, Nguyen M, Campbell S (1999) Doppler fetal circulation in pregnancies complicated by pre-eclampsia or delivery of a small for gestational age baby: 2. Longitudinal analysis. *Br J Obstet Gynaecol* **106**(5), 453–66.

Hecher K, Campbell S (1996) Characteristics of fetal venous blood flow under normal circumstances and during fetal disease. *Ultrasound Obstet Gynecol* **7**(1), 68–83.

8

CASE HISTORIES AND SCENARIOS

1. ABNORMAL UTERINE ARTERY DOPPLER AND NORMAL FETAL GROWTH AT 24 WEEKS

Screening for pre-eclampsia and intrauterine growth retardation (IUGR) is best performed at 20–24 weeks. If bilateral uterine artery notches are seen, or there is raised uterine artery resistance, it is unusual (though not rare) for fetal growth already to be impaired or fetal arterial redistribution to be seen. Those women in whom early onset IUGR occurs are more likely to be those with a previous poor obstetric history, or those with essential hypertension, cardiac or renal conditions or antiphospholipid syndrome.

The Doppler images in Fig. 8.1 show deep bilateral notches with high impedance at 24 weeks. This is a particularly high-risk combination. In this scan, there is normal fetal growth, activity and amniotic fluid; arterial Dopplers are also normal.

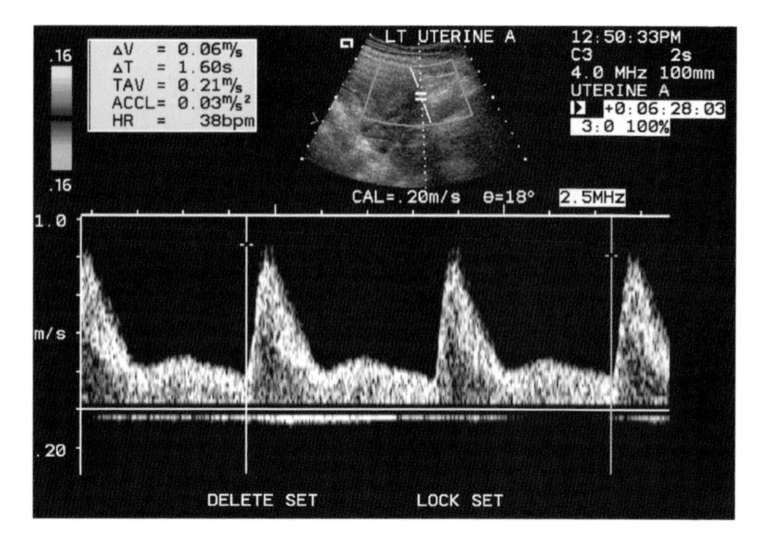

Figure 8.1(a) Bilateral uterine artery notches/high resistance waveforms. Left uterine artery.

The positive predictive value for adverse outcome (pre-eclampsia, IUGR, placental abruption or stillbirth) is greater than 50% in these women. In this particular case, it is suggested that women are counseled with the following key pieces of information:

- There is impaired uteroplacental Doppler
- Fetal growth, amniotic fluid and umbilical artery Doppler are normal
- There is an increased risk of pre-eclampsia and/or delivering a baby that is small for gestation
- It is recommended that a scan for fetal growth is repeated every 3 weeks
- It is suggested that maternal blood pressure is checked and urinalysis performed at least every 2 weeks

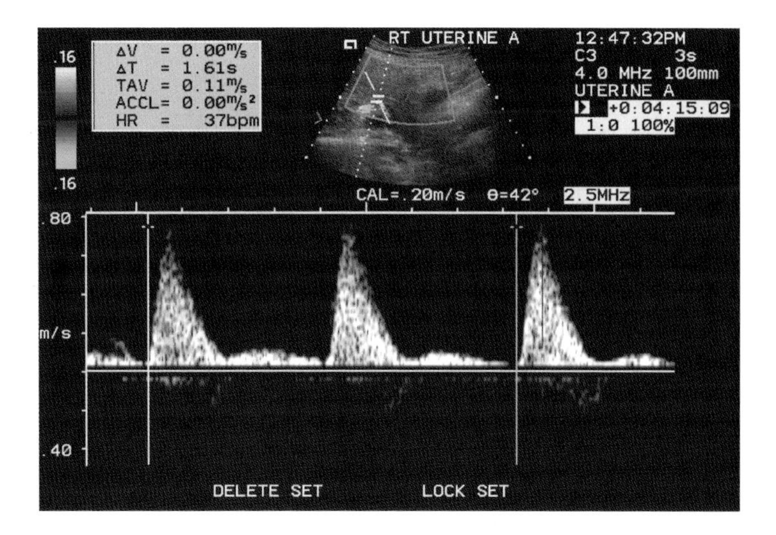

Figure 8.1(b) The very poor end-diastolic flow in the right uterine artery waveform almost hides the notch.

It is possible to provide individual likelihood ratios for severe adverse pregnancy outcome on the basis of mean uterine artery Doppler pulsatility index (PI) at 23 weeks. This chart is shown in Appendix B.

2. BILATERAL UTERINE ARTERY NOTCHES AND FETAL GROWTH REDUCING

The patient was at 27 weeks, the first recall following the 24-week screening scan. Fetal growth had reduced to the 10th percentile. Although amniotic fluid and fetal movements are normal, there is increased umbilical artery resistance (feto-placental Doppler) with absent umbilical end-diastolic flow (EDF) (Fig. 8.2). The middle

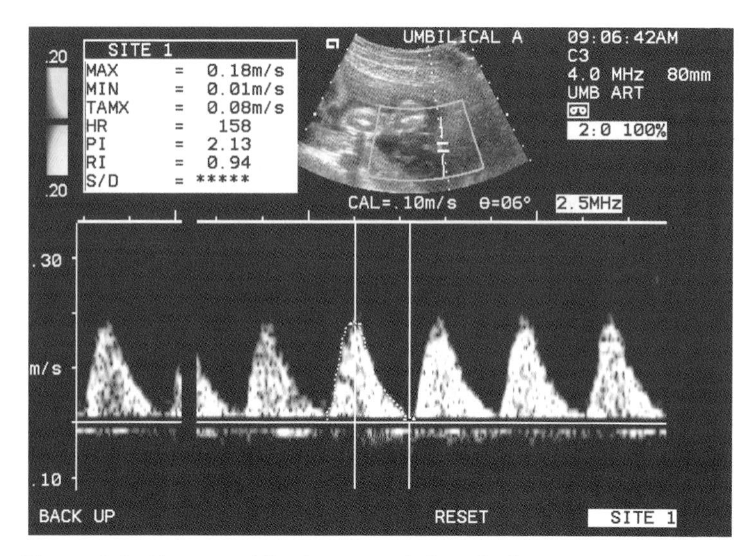

Figure 8.2 Absent umbilical artery end-diastolic flow, with pulsatility index (PI) > 95th percentile.

cerebral artery (MCA) Doppler shows increased EDF (Fig. 8.3), although the ductus venous waveform remains normal (Fig. 8.4). At this stage, a cardiotocograph (CTG) is performed (Fig. 8.5), maternal steroid administration is advised and a joint obstetric/neonatal review undertaken. The decision for delivery depends on the rate at which fetal deterioration occurs, or whether pre-eclampsia supervenes. Delivery is usually within 1–4 weeks.

Follow-up

A reasonable plan would be to rescan weekly for growth and fetal arterial Dopplers. Blood pressure/urinalysis should be checked weekly.

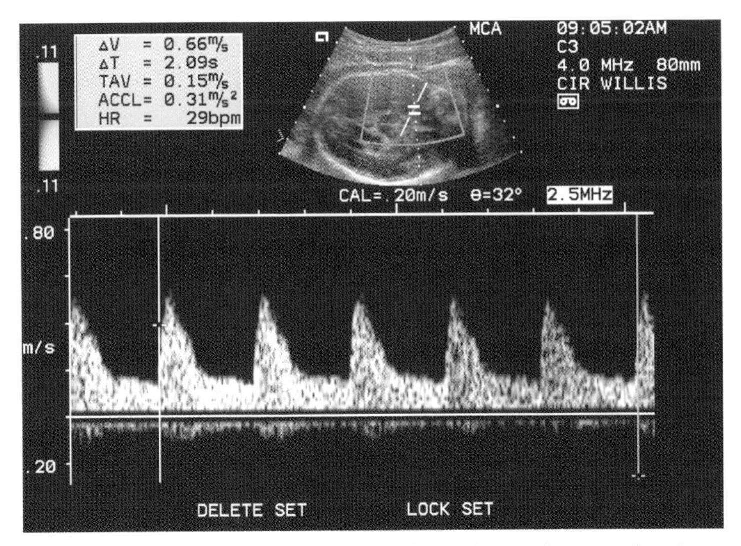

Figure 8.3 Middle cerebral artery waveform showing increased end-diastolic flow consistent with a brain-sparing effect.

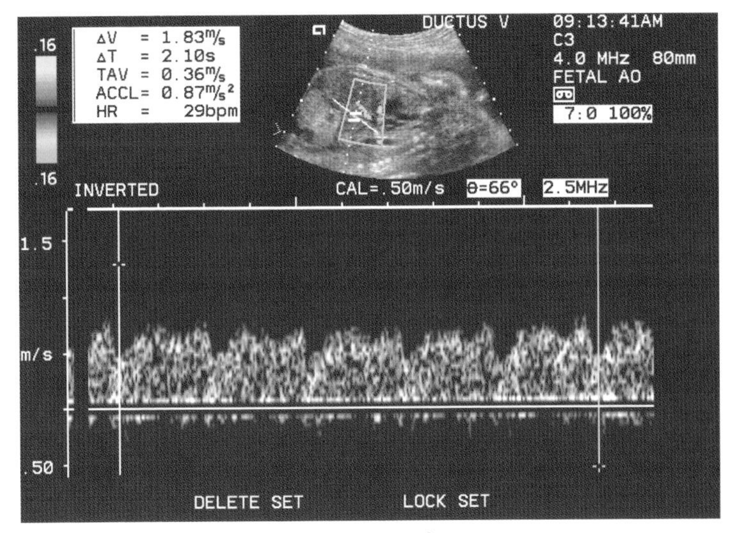

Figure 8.4 Normal ductus venosus waveform.

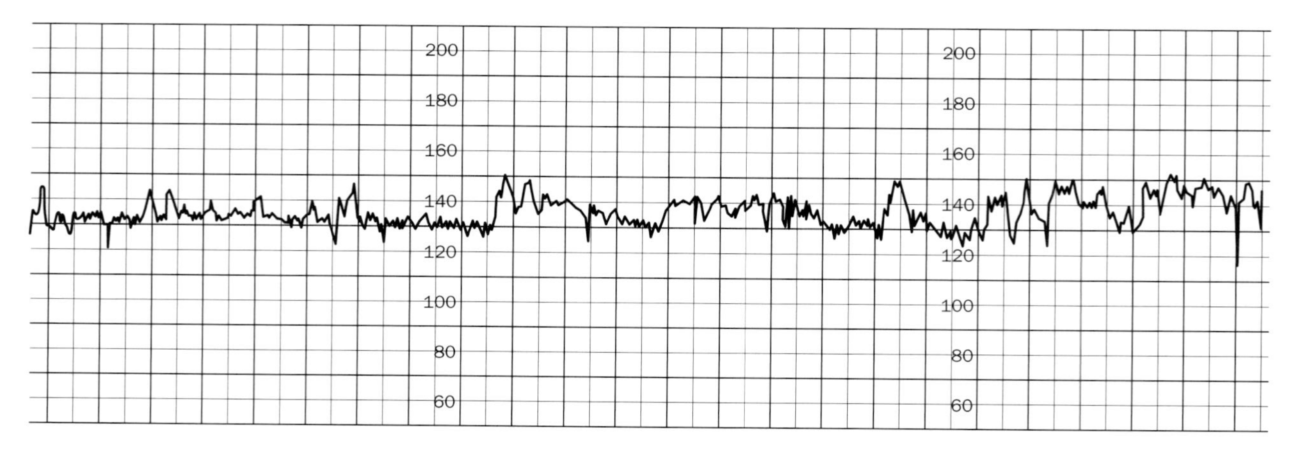

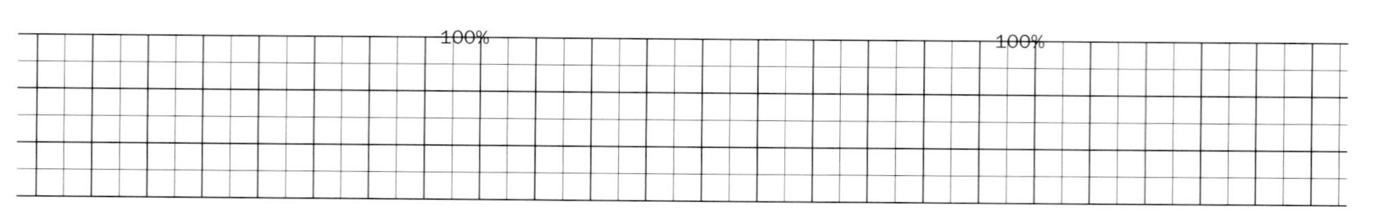

Figure 8.5 Normal cardiotocograph showing good variability and the presence of accelerations.

3. FETAL GROWTH RESTRICTION WITH ARTERIAL REDISTRIBUTION AND VENOUS CHANGES

This patient presented for routine Doppler follow up at 29 weeks' gestation. Three weeks prior to this appointment there was normal fetal growth and all was well, except for the presence of bilateral uterine artery notches.

There is severe growth restriction (Fig. 8.6). Not only is there severe arterial redistribution (Fig. 8.7), but the fetal heart is visibly enlarged with poor contractility and the bowel is hyperechogenic. The ductus venosus Doppler is clearly abnormal with an exaggerated 'a' wave. The CTG (Fig. 8.8) shows unprovoked decelerations and reduced variability. This fetus has a high probability of intrauterine demise within 48 h if not delivered.

Follow-up

Further Doppler surveillance is of only academic value. Unless there are major fetal or maternal reasons why delivery is to be delayed (fetus previable, no available neonatal cot and *in-utero* transfer not possible because of maternal condition), delivery should be expedited within 24–48 h.

Outcome

A classical Caesarean section was undertaken within 2 h of these findings and a 740 g male baby was delivered. The mother developed severe postpartum pre-eclampsia requiring intravenous antihypertensive medication and prophylactic anticonvulsants.

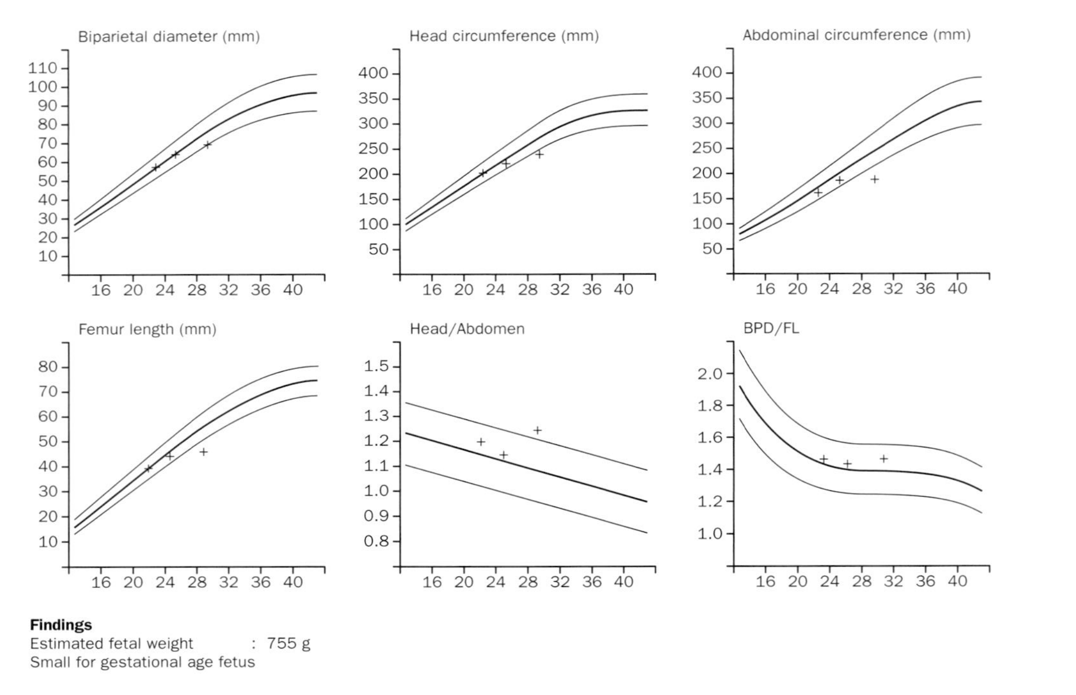

Figure 8.6 Biometry charts showing a reduction in growth velocity and an increase in the head circumference–abdomen circumference ratio.

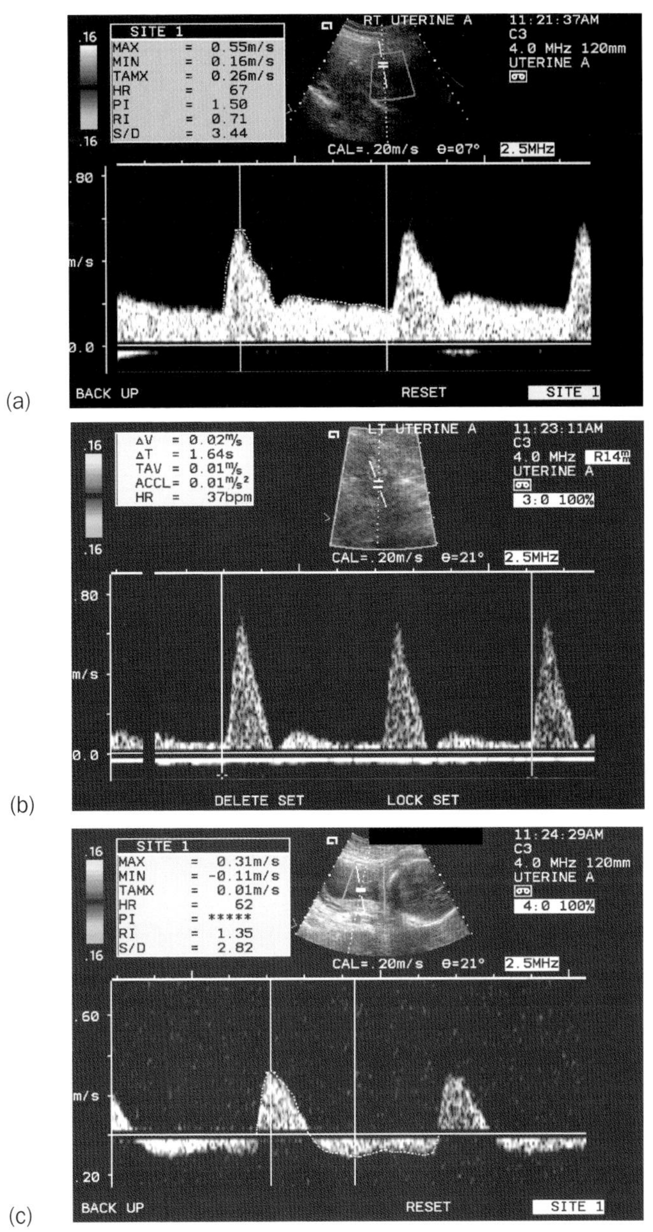

Figure 8.7 The waveforms in (a) and (b) show bilateral uterine artery notches. Reverse end-diastolic flow in the umbilical artery is shown in (c).

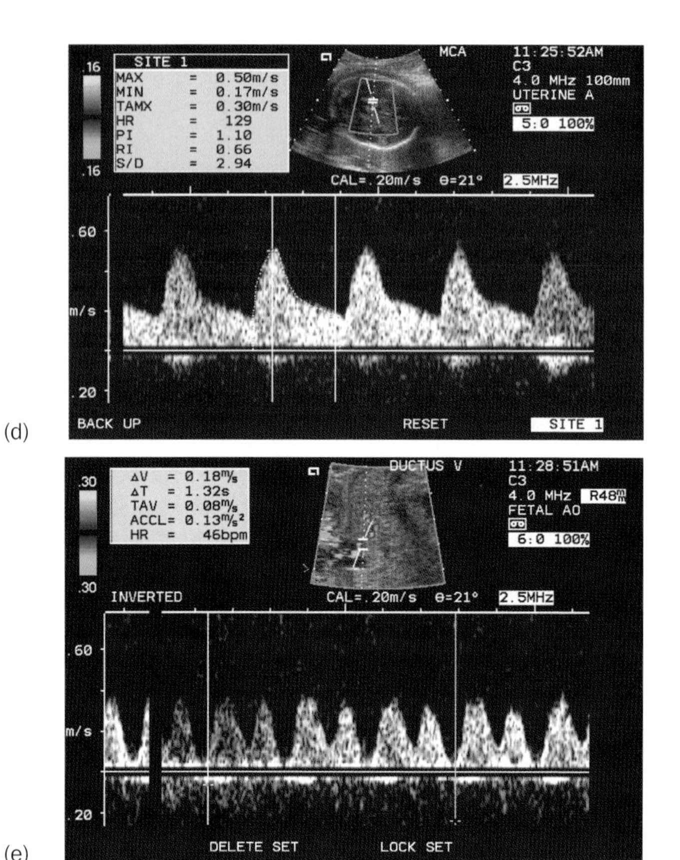

Figure 8.7 (*continued*) (d) shows brain-sparing in the middle cerebral artery. The ductus venosus with an 'a' wave reaching the baseline is shown in (e).

4. PHYSIOLOGICAL ARTERIAL REDISTRIBUTION AT TERM

As the fetus becomes more mature (after 34 weeks), deoxygenated blood passing though the left atrium and ventricle is preferentially directed to the brain at the expense of oxygenated blood. This leads to 'physiological' brain-sparing (Fig. 8.9). Middle cerebral artery

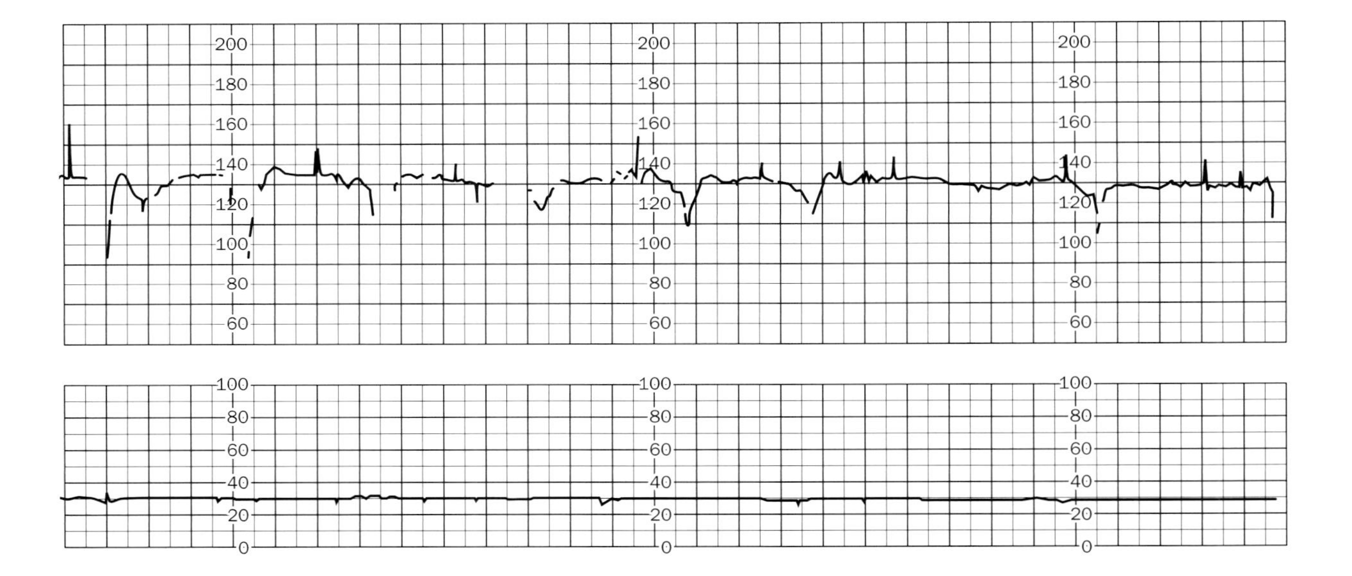

Figure 8.8 Cardiotocograph showing reduced variability, absent accelerations and unprovoked decelerations.

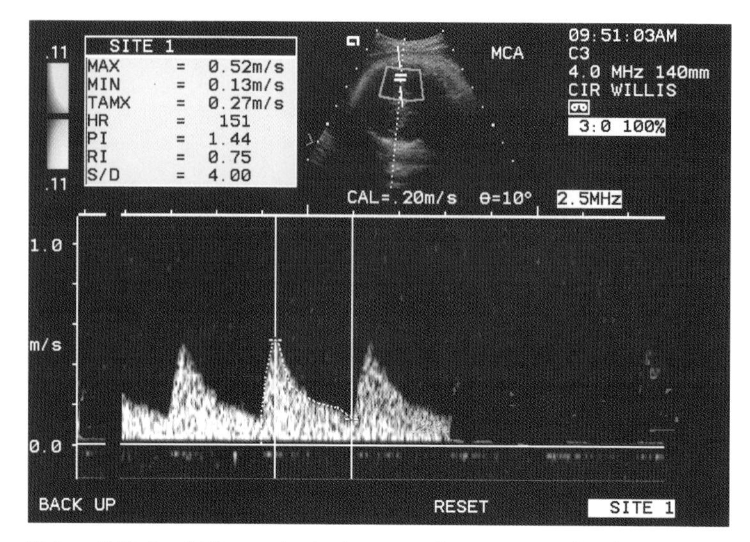

Figure 8.9 A middle cerebral artery waveform at term showing extensive end-diastolic flow, implying physiological redistribution.

flow, which might be considered pathological at earlier stages of gestation, is quite normal at this stage.

After 34 weeks, umbilical artery Doppler becomes unreliable in that false-negatives may occur. At this stage of gestation, as a result of the high umbilical arterial velocities, a very considerable increase in feto-placental impedance is required for umbilical artery Doppler to become abnormal. This means that one cannot rely solely on 'reduced or absent EDF' in the umbilical artery at these later gestations. This effect, combined with anomalous MCA flow, means that arterial Dopplers after 34 weeks require very careful interpretation. This is one occasion when the thoracic aorta and ductus venosus Doppler, although technically difficult to measure because of fetal size and position, will often provide vital extra information.

5. FETAL ANEMIA

Rhesus iso-immunization may lead to fetal anemia, through maternal antibodies passing into the fetal circulation causing red

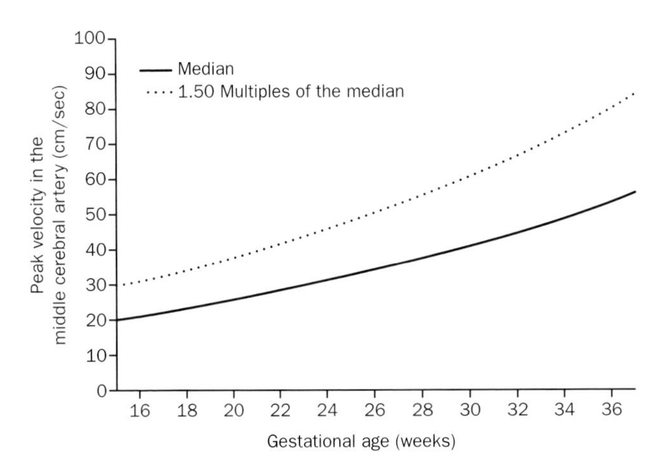

Figure 8.10 Middle cerebral artery peak systolic velocity related to gestational age. After Mari, G, Deter, RL, Carpenter, RL et al. Non-invasive diagnosis by Doppler ultrasonography of fetal anaemia due to maternal red-cell alloimmunization. *N Engl J Med* **432**(1), 9–14, Figure 3.

blood cell destruction. This, in turn, will lead to greater fetal cardiac output, a hyperdynamic circulation and increased velocity of blood flowing through arterial vessels. This phenomenon allows fetal anemia to be monitored non-invasively using Doppler. Peak systolic velocity of the MCA correlates well with the degree of fetal anemia, allowing a more precise decision as to when fetal blood sampling is carried out. Serial measurements may be made in the same woman over the course of many weeks (see Fig 8.10).

6. FETAL ANEMIA CAUSED BY RHESUS DISEASE WITH CARDIAC FAILURE

As discussed above, a severely anemic fetus will have a hyperdynamic circulation. The heart will be enlarged and this is often associated with a pericardial effusion. Arterial Dopplers may show increased velocities, particularly in the cerebral circulation. In late anemia with fetal hydrops, venous return to the fetal heart

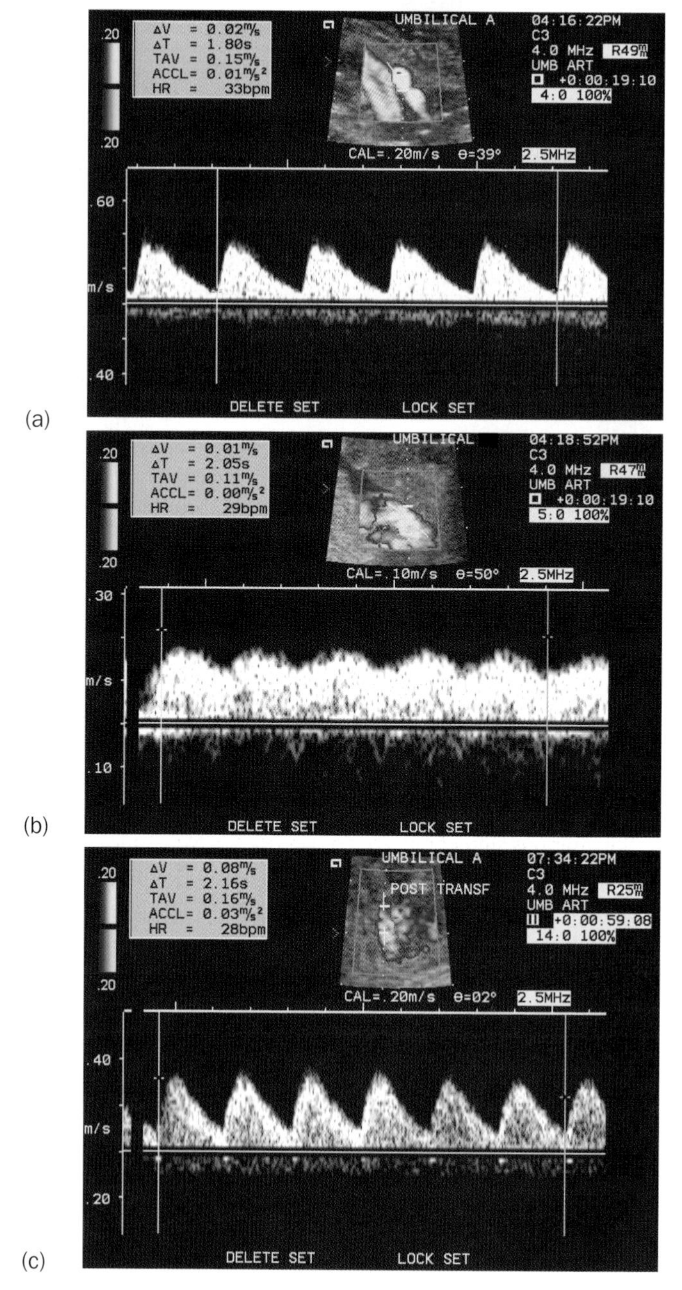

Figure 8.11 The waveforms show a normal pre-transfusion umbilical artery Doppler (a) waveform with, in (b), abnormal umbilical venous pulsations. The post-transfusion waveforms show no change in the umbilical artery waveform (c).

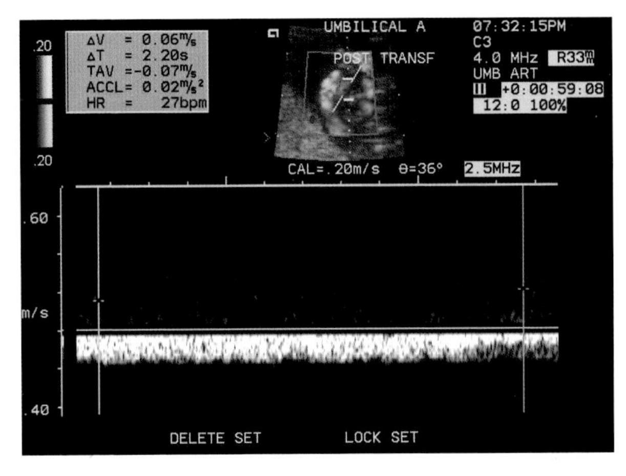

Figure 8.11 (*continued*) The post-transfusion umbilical venous waveform is now normal (d), showing a 'reversal' of cardiac failure.

is impaired, which may be indicated by umbilical venous pulsations and 'a'-wave reversal in the ductus venosus.

Figure 8.11 illustrates the reversal of cardiac failure following intrauterine intravascular blood transfusion. The umbilical vein, which showed the ominous sign of pulsations, has normalized following blood administration, indicating an improvement in cardiac function. Umbilical artery Doppler, as expected, remains unchanged throughout.

FURTHER READING

Mari G, Deter RL, Carpenter RL, Rahman F, Zimmerman R, Moise KJ Jr, et al. (2000) Noninvasive diagnosis by Doppler ultrasonography of fetal anemia due to maternal red-cell alloimmunization. Collaborative Group for Doppler Assessment of the Blood Velocity in Anemic Fetuses. *N Engl J Med* **342**(1), 9–14.

APPENDIX A

PULSED-WAVE DOPPLER ULTRASOUND VELOCITY MEASUREMENT

Color-flow and pulsed-wave Doppler images are derived from measurement of movement between pulses.

Figure A.1 shows a scatterer in blood moving through a beam of ultrasound. Ultrasound is scattered from red blood cells although the back-scattering from blood is complex and depends on many factors, including shear rate, hematocrit and local fluctuations in red blood cell density.

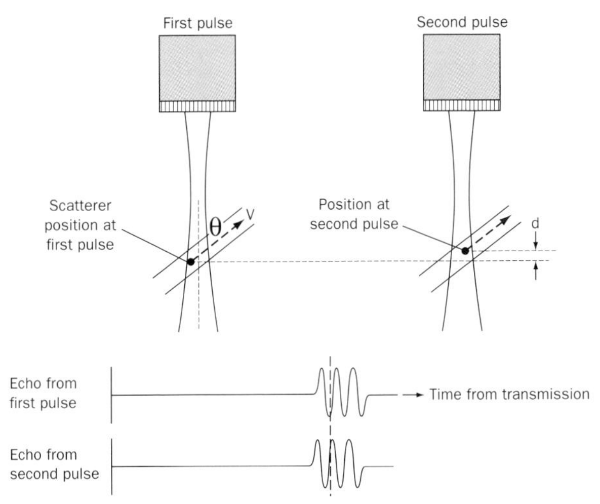

Figure A.1 Ultrasound detection of blood flow. The transmit-to-receive time of the returning echo from a moving scatterer changes from pulse to pulse as its position in the beam changes. In this case, the scatterer is slightly nearer to the transducer when the second pulse is transmitted and the echo arrives back at the transducer earlier than it did for the first.

Pulses of ultrasound are sent at a pulse repetition frequency (PRF). In Fig. A.1, the distance moved between pulses in the direction of the beam (d) is measured. By determining the angle between the direction of movement and the beam (θ) the velocity (V) along the vessel can be calculated by:

$$V = d \times \text{PRF} \times \frac{1}{\cos\theta}$$

As can be seen from the two returning echoes in Fig. A.1, the echo from the second pulse returns slightly sooner than the first because the scatterer is now nearer the transducer. The change in transmit-to-receive time can be used to measure the distance moved. Alternatively, at a particular time, the phase of the returned echo will be different. Phase-shift can be described as the change in angle of two cyclic signals. For example, in Fig. A.2 the two signals on the left are in phase and the two on the right are 90° (more usually written as $\pi/2$ radians) out of phase.

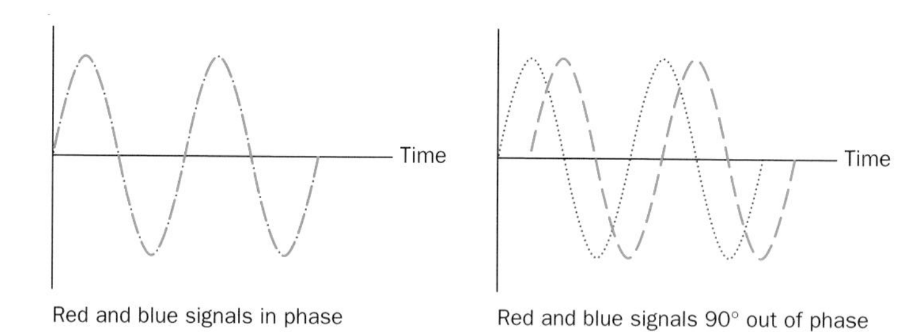

Figure A.2 Two signals (red and blue) in (left) and out of (right) phase.

Figure A.3 shows how the Doppler signal is obtained. The upper traces show the phase of two consecutive echoes at a point in time following transmission (blue dotted line). The phase change, ϕ, is a measure of the distance the scatterer has travelled along the beam because it is a fraction of the wavelength of the transmitted ultrasound:

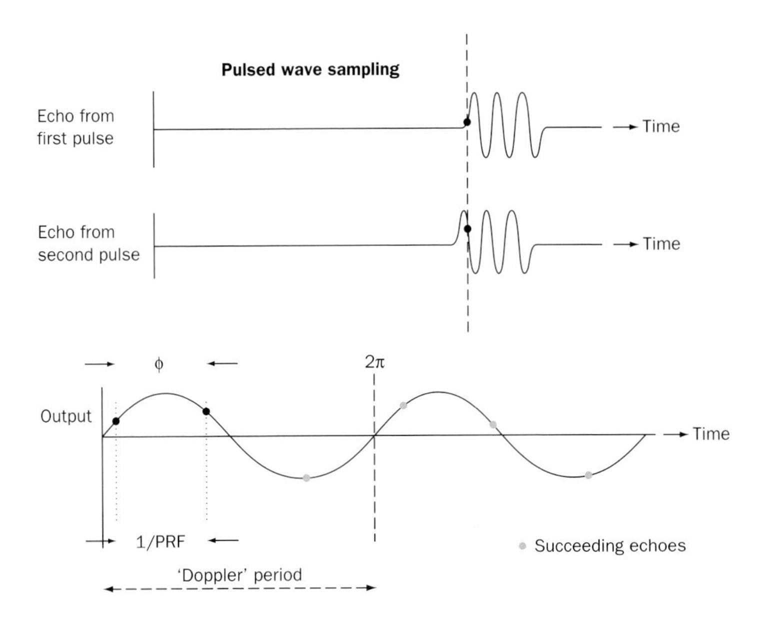

Figure A.3 Measurement of the change in phase of the returning signals produces the Doppler frequency (lower) line.

$$d = \frac{\phi}{2\pi} \times \frac{c}{f_t} \times \frac{1}{2}$$

Distance = fraction of complete cycle × wavelength divided by two, since the transmit-to-scattering and scattering-to-receive times are identically reduced.

The velocity is now (combining the first two equations):

$$V = \frac{\phi}{2\pi} \times \frac{c}{f_t} \times \frac{\text{PRF}}{2\cos\theta}$$

The change in phase with each pulse gives rise to what is commonly referred to as the Doppler frequency (f_d) (Fig. A.3, lower trace), which is dependent on the phase change and PRF as follows:

$$f_d = \frac{\phi}{2\pi} \times \text{PRF}$$

Combining the last two equations gives

$$V = \frac{f_d c}{2 f_t \cos\theta}$$

which is more usually written as

$$f_d = \frac{2 V f_t \cos\theta}{c}$$

(the Doppler equation).

In practice, the Doppler output is very complex and will contain many frequencies as a result of the many velocities in the sample volume and the complex interaction of the pulse scattering from the blood.

In **pulsed-wave** Doppler displays, a Fourier analysis is used to display the range of frequencies in a sonogram (the spectral display).

In **color-flow** image mapping, autocorrelation methods determine the mean and variance of the phase shift to produce a value for the motion in the direction of the beam which is displayed as a color pixel.

ALIASING

The rate at which the moving scatterers are sampled is critical to the performance of the flow-imaging modes. The movement is sampled at a PRF, as described above.

For low velocities, a low PRF is used to detect the small movement between pulses. If too high a PRF is used, the relative motion between pulses may not be detected. However, low PRFs can give rise to problems when sampling high velocities. The effect is shown in Fig. A.4, where the scatterer moves so far between pulses that the phase change measured is incorrect.

The first echo registers a phase from the first cycle of the pulse. The second echo records a phase from the second cycle in the pulse. The processor is unable to discriminate and so registers the movement (and therefore velocity) as a change in phase of the same cycle leading to an erroneous f_d:

$$f_d = \frac{\phi}{2\pi} \times \text{PRF}$$

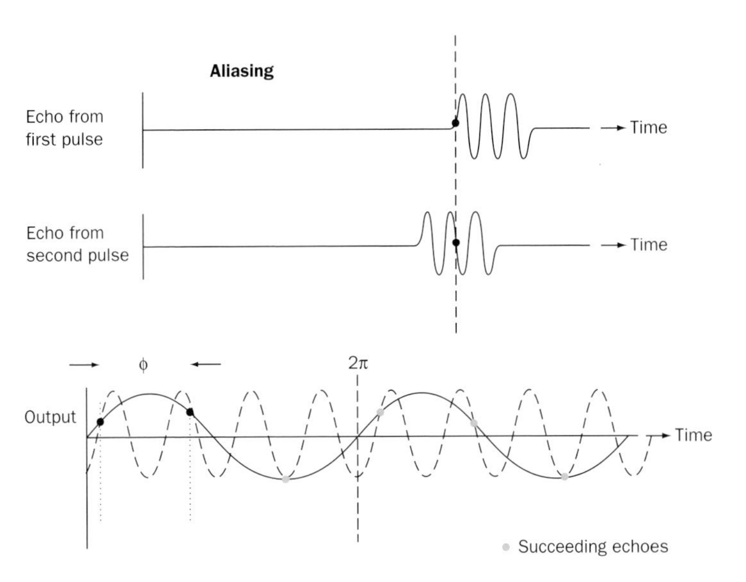

Figure A.4 Inadequate sampling of the change in phase produces an incorrect Doppler frequency (solid black line) and leads to aliasing. The true frequency is shown by the dotted blue line.

(solid line in Fig. A.4), whereas the true f_d is

$$f_d = \frac{2\pi + \phi}{2\pi} \times \text{PRF}$$

(dashed line in Fig. A.4)

ALIASING AND PULSED DOPPLER LIMITS

In order to measure the correct 'Doppler' frequency, the PRF must be at least twice the Doppler frequency. If the PRF is too low, an erroneous Doppler frequency will result (Fig. A.4). This is sometimes referred to as the Nyquist limit.

The PRF itself is limited by the need for a pulse to travel to the sample volume and back before a second pulse is transmitted. If a second pulse is transmitted before the first is received, there will be a range ambiguity with echoes from a deep sample volume from the first pulse and a shallow sample volume from the second. To avoid this, the maximum PRF is limited so that an unambiguous sample volume gate is used. Since it takes longer for the pulse to make its return trip from deeper sample volumes than from shallow tissue, the maximum PRF is reduced with increasing depth. This in turn limits the maximum Doppler frequency and velocity that can be measured at depth. This can be calculated by:

$$f_{d\,\text{max}} = \frac{\text{PRF}}{2}$$

$$\text{PRF} = \frac{c}{2d}$$

where c is the speed of sound in tissue and d is the depth of the sample volume. Combining these gives

$$f_{d\,\text{max}} = \frac{c}{4d}$$

and putting this in the Doppler equation gives

$$f_{d\ max} = \frac{2\,V_{max}\,f_t\cos\theta}{c}$$

$$V_{max}\,d\,\cos\theta = \frac{c^2}{8\,f_t}$$

In practice, this maximum velocity can be extended by a factor of two by moving the baseline (by assuming that flow is unidirectional) but is has three important practical implications for PW ultrasound:

- Maximum velocity measurable **decreases** with depth
- Maximum velocity measurable **decreases** the more aligned the beam is to flow
- Maximum velocity measurable **increases** with a lower transmit frequency

APPENDIX B

LIKELIHOOD RATIO FOR SEVERE ADVERSE OUTCOME RELATING TO MEAN UTERINE PULSATILITY INDEX AT 23 WEEKS

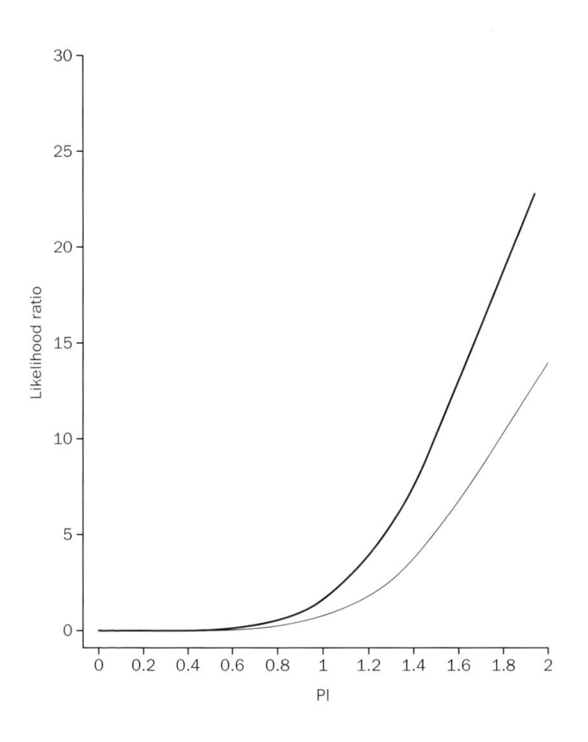

Figure B.1 The likelihood ratio for severe adverse outcome, namely pre-eclampsia before 34 weeks, small for gestation delivery < 10th percentile before 34 weeks, placental abruption and fetal death related to mean pulsatility index (PI). Smokers are represented by a thick black line, non-smokers by a thin line. Figure reproduced with permission from the American College of Obstetricians and Gynecologists (*Obstetrics and Gynecology*, 2001 **98**(3), 369–73).

APPENDIX C

FETAL ARTERIAL AND VENOUS PULSATILITY INDEX AND TIME-AVERAGED VELOCITY CHARTS

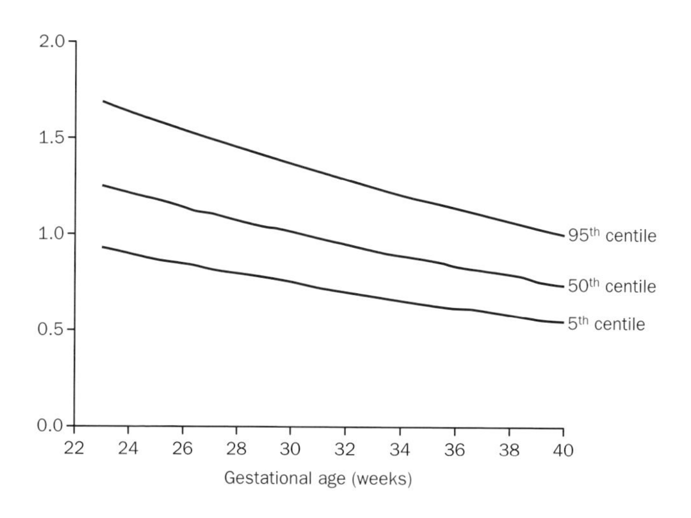

Figure C.1 Umbilical artery pulsatility index (Parra, Lees et al., unpublished).

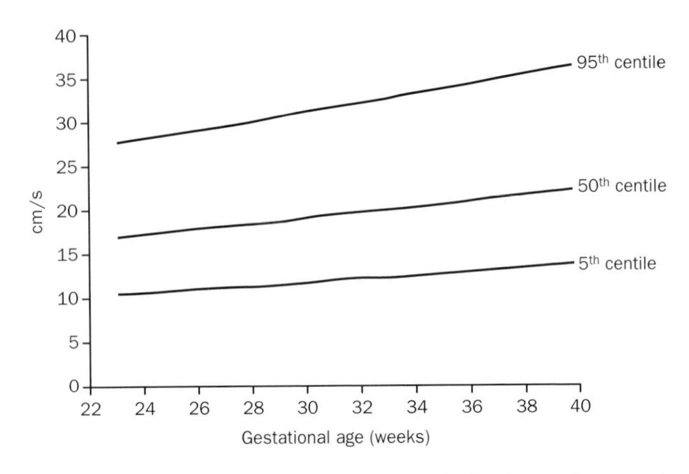

Figure C.2 Umbilical artery time-averaged velocity (Parra, Lees et al., unpublished).

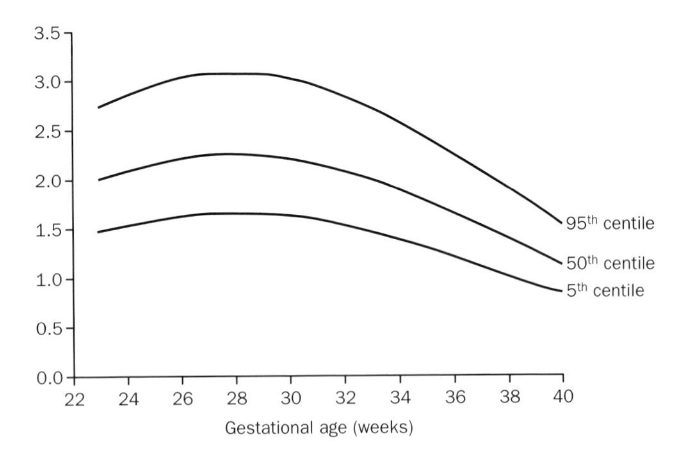

Figure C.3 Middle cerebral artery pulsatility index (Parra, Lees et al., unpublished).

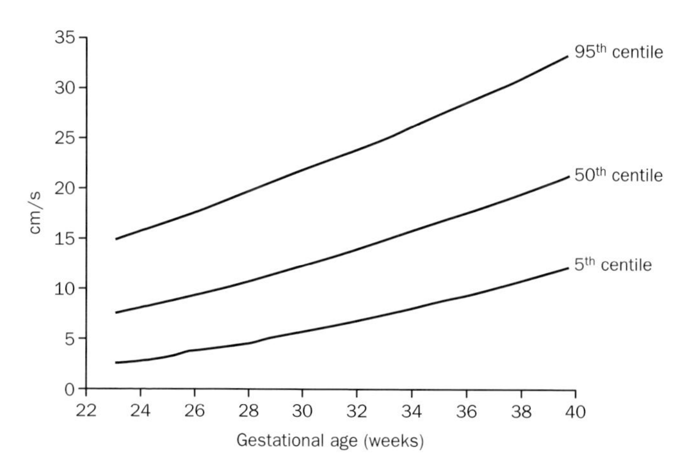

Figure C.4 Middle cerebral artery time-averaged velocity (Parra, Lees et al., unpublished).

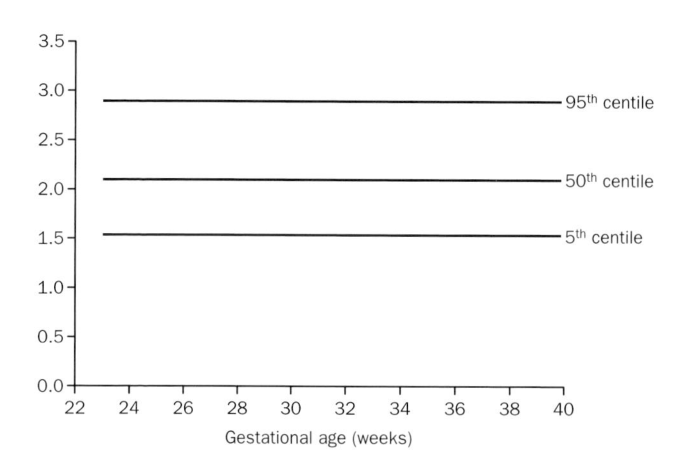

Figure C.5 Thoracic aorta pulsatility index (Parra, Lees et al., unpublished).

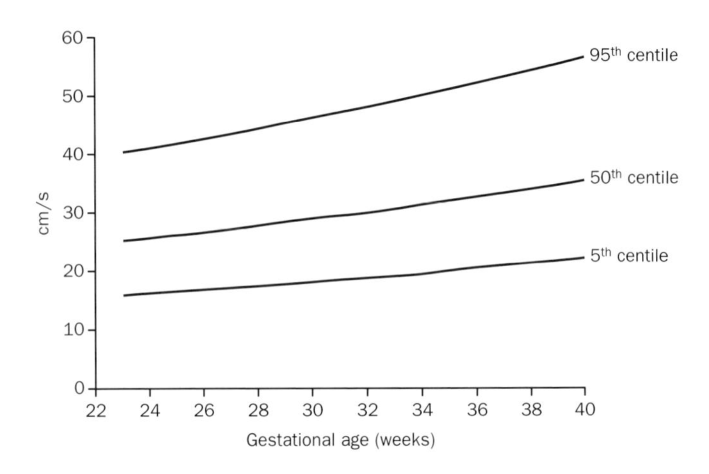

Figure C.6 Thoracic aorta time-averaged velocity (Parra, Lees et al., unpublished).

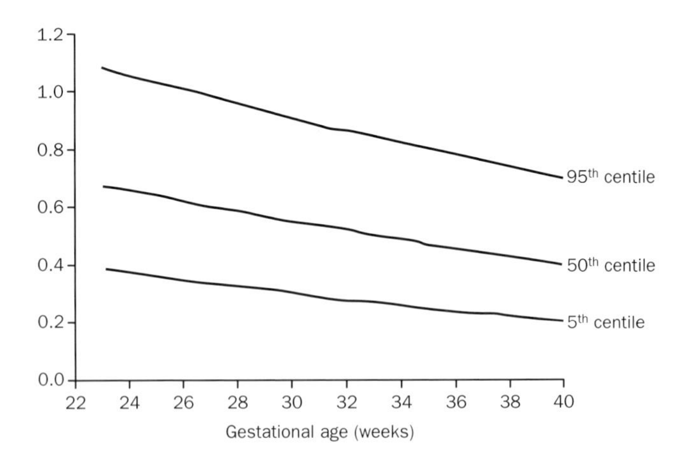

Figure C.7 Ductus venosus pulsatility index (Parra, Lees et al., unpublished).

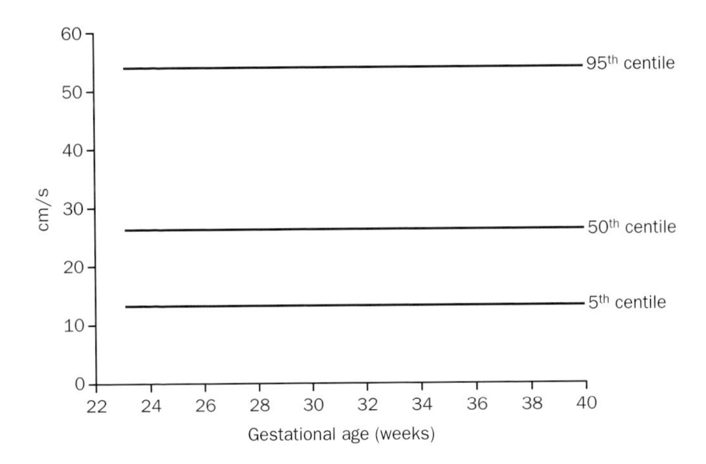

Figure C.8 Ductus venosus time-averaged velocity (Parra, Lees et al., unpublished).

INDEX

Page numbers in *italics* refer to figures and tables.